GETTING INTO MEDICAL SCHOOL TODAY

Scott H. Plantz, M.D.
with
Nicholas Y. Lorenzo, M.D.
Jesse A. Cole, M.D.

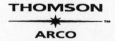

Australia • Canada • Mexico • Singapore • Spain • United Kingdom • United States

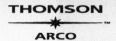

THOMSON

ARCO

For my mother, Pauline Christensen Plantz,
without whose support this book could not
have been written.

For more information, contact Peterson's, 2000 Lenox Drive, Lawrenceville, NJ 08648; 800-338-3282; or find us on the World Wide Web at www.petersons.com/about.

Fourth Edition

Library of Congress Number: 97-81127

ISBN: 0-02-862500-5

Printed in Canada

10 9 8 7 6   06 05 04

CONTENTS

FOREWORD v

ABOUT THE AUTHORS vi

ACKNOWLEDGMENTS vii

  1. MEDICINE AS A CAREER 1

  2. HIGH SCHOOL PREPARATION AND
      COLLEGE SELECTION 9

  3. COLLEGE PROFESSORS/ADVISORS 15

  4. FRESHMAN CLASSES 21

  5. MAJOR SELECTION 27

  6. CORE REQUIREMENTS 33

  7. SCIENCE GRADE MAINTENANCE 35

  8. STUDY HABITS 41

  9. PART-TIME JOBS 47

10. COLLEGE ACTIVITIES 53

11. APPLICATION FORMS 59

12. THE MEDICAL COLLEGE ADMISSION TEST 77

13. LETTERS OF RECOMMENDATION 81

14. CURRICULUM VITAE PREPARATION 87

15. WHERE TO APPLY 93

16. INTERVIEWS 97

17. MEDICAL SCHOOL SELECTION AND FINANCIAL AID ... 105

18. SPECIAL APPLICANTS: MINORITIES, OLDER STUDENTS, AND WOMEN 115

19. WHAT TO DO IF YOU DO NOT GET IN 123

20. MEDICAL SCHOOL 135

21. RESIDENCY 145

22. GOALS, PRIORITIES, AND CONCLUSIONS 155

APPENDIX: ACCREDITED U.S. MEDICAL SCHOOLS 157

FOREWORD

Getting Into Medical School Today is a new, up-to-date book all students considering a medical career should read. The authors have adopted a no-nonsense, step-by-step approach premedical students can follow to reach their career goals. The book provides detailed "do's" and "don'ts" of high school and college preparation for a medical career. Most important, it helps students avoid the pitfalls and negotiate the stumbling blocks they may encounter early in their college years.

The authors dispel many of the romantic ideas not only about how to get into medical school, but about what medical school itself entails. This book is pragmatic. Several chapters are devoted to topics such as how to prepare for college and select college courses and instructors. For the student lacking an experienced premedical advisor, this book fills the gap, providing sound recommendations on selecting an appropriate curriculum for completing a premedical education. The authors pull no punches; they emphasize both the work required and the "games" that must be played to make one's way to medical school acceptance. Detailed chapters discuss such issues as completing application forms, preparing for the MCAT, obtaining letters of recommendation, selecting medical schools, and preparing for medical school interviews. They also address practical issues like housing and financial aid.

Nothing I have read could be more practical, realistic, or useful for high school or college students contemplating a medical career.

Marion Sitzmann, Ph.D., O.S.B.
Professor of English and Speech
Premedical Advisor, Creighton University

About the Authors

Scott H. Plantz, M.D., born in Hastings, Nebraska, is currently the Research Director at the Department of Emergency Medicine, Mt. Sinai Medical Center, Chicago, Illinois, and Assistant Professor of Emergency Medicine at Chicago Medical School. He is also Vice-President of the American Academy of Emergency Medicine. He completed his residency in emergency medicine at Rush–Presbyterian's Emergency Medicine residency program at Christ Hospital, Oak Lawn, Illinois. Prior to his residency, he completed his internship at Michigan State University's Emergency Medicine program at Butterworth Hospital, Grand Rapids, Michigan. He graduated from the University of Nebraska College of Medicine and was a Summa Cum Laude graduate of Creighton University in Omaha, Nebraska.

Nicholas Y. Lorenzo, M.D., is a native of Albany, New York, who now calls Kansas City, Kansas, home. He is currently an ophthalmology resident at the University of Kansas. Prior to his residency in Kansas, Dr. Lorenzo completed a residency in neurology in the Department of Neurology at the Mayo Clinic, Rochester, Minnesota. Prior to his fellowship he completed an internal medicine internship at the Mayo Clinic. Dr. Lorenzo graduated with High Distinction from the University of Nebraska College of Medicine and is a member of the Alpha Omega Alpha Honor Medical Society. He is a Magna Cum Laude graduate of Creighton University.

Jesse A. Cole, M.D., born in Cheyenne, Wyoming, is a Magna Cum Laude graduate of Augustana College. Dr. Cole completed his medical training at Creighton University and is a member of the Alpha Omega Honor Medical Society. He completed his residency training in radiology at St. Louis University. He also completed a fellowship in immunology at the National Institute of Health and is currently in private practice in Billings, Montana.

ACKNOWLEDGMENTS

I have been learning all my life. Almost every individual I have met has taught me something. Teachers taught me facts that I occasionally remember but most often forget. Administrators taught me to accept red tape as a fact of life. Some of the information I have acquired has come from successful students who taught me how they overcame a very selective system. The most important information I have learned came from observing students who did not reach their goals.

Special thanks to Randolph P. Scott, Pharm.D., M.D., Ph.D., a master at getting around the system. To Phillip R. Hynes, M.D., whose ability to overcome severe setbacks is inspirational. To my close friend Jesse A. Cole, M.D., whose level-headedness has continued to provide a stabilizing influence on my life. For their loyal support: Nicholas Y. Lorenzo, M.D.; Ed Arevalo, M.D.; Jenifer Arevalo, M.A.; Julie Overcash, M.D.; Cliff O'Callahan, Ph.D., M.D.; Rebecca Schmidt, M.A.; Jeffrey Meade, M.D.; Theodore Yee, M.D.; Wayne Wolfrey, M.D.; and Jeffrey Rapp, M.D., whose friendship made medical school a tolerable experience. To my friends Charles Boehrer, J.D., Paul Crawford, J.D., Joseph Vandenack, J.D., Bruce Bohlen, Daniel Kerr, Steve Marvel, Pam Martin, and Mark Janssen, who stuck by me when the going got tough.

Several instructors made a difference in my education, not only because they were excellent teachers, but because they were people I strove to emulate. Three high school instructors are especially noteworthy: the late Dale Feeken, Donald Retzlaff, and Patty Olsen, who taught me respectively to think, to be organized, and to speak in public. Special thanks to my two premedical advisors and friends, the late Father Marion Sitzmann, Ph.D., and Douglas Lund, Ph.D., each of whom recommended me for medical school. To the late Harold Heaston, C.P.A., the most challenging instructor I have ever had. Finally, thanks to my neuroanatomy instructor, the late Professor Alvin Earle, Ph.D., whose kindness and friendship made medical school a survivable experience.

Most of all, I thank my parents, Alan and Pauline Plantz, and brother, Brad, who taught me that success in life requires hard work, perseverance, tolerance, confidence, and luck, and that holding onto that success requires much, much more.

Scott H. Plantz, M.D.

MEDICINE AS A CAREER

**"It's what you learn after you know
it all that counts."**

Harry S. Truman

"It's your first day in the emergency room as the intern on call. Standing in your freshly pressed white coat, idly chatting with the nurses as you prescribe treatment for your first patient of the day, a child with an ear infection, you feel on top of the world, elated at having made the diagnosis (and forgetting the nurse's opening statement on presenting you the chart, 'I think he has an ear infection') and grateful to know the treatment without sneaking off to look it up. Suddenly, the doors burst open and two ambulance attendants wheel in a blood-soaked pile of clothing strapped to a backboard. It looks as if it has two arms and legs but you're not sure. 'He can't breathe!' one paramedic shouts as they quickly transfer it (you're still not sure if there's a human being in the mess, much less a man or a woman) to the gurney.

"As the curtains are drawn around the trauma area and two nurses rush to start intravenous lines and draw blood, a single thought screams into your mind and you narrowly miss biting your tongue, teeth clenching to prevent the words from escaping: 'Somebody get a doctor!'"

Most physicians would agree that selecting medicine as a career should be a very difficult process. Many of them, however, acknowledge that medicine seems to have selected them.

1

Medicine offers an exciting, challenging, and rewarding career; it also requires the longest and most extensive training of any of the professions. As a physician you will assume the role of a healer, confidant, and role model for the community in which you live. A doctor's influential position is noteworthy, but it is not without sacrifice. Your time will never again be your own and your personal life will constantly be scrutinized by the people in your community.

TRAINING

Becoming a physician merely begins with the completion of medical school. Its achievement is a lifelong task. Training will dominate some of the best years of your life. In addition to your high school education, you will spend three to four years in college. As a college student, you will be required to take several difficult science courses and your overall performance must be good to excellent in the classes you take. While your friends are enjoying the social events of the week, you will be making yet another trip to the library.

Medical school is not fun and games. If you thought college was difficult, look out! The phrase "Medical school is like trying to take a sip from a fire hydrant" is quoted often for good reason. Medical school at most institutions requires four years. The first two years will make your college courses seem easy, as you will be required to take 24 to 28 hours of rigorous science classes per semester. A frequent description of the first two years is "The material is not really that difficult, it's just the never-ending volume that makes the whole process a challenge." The final two years of clinical sciences are much more enjoyable. Although the time commitment is substantial, you will finally have a role in direct patient management.

Residency is a minimum of three to four years after medical school for most medical specialties including family practice, pediatrics, internal medicine, neurology, emergency medicine, obstetrics and gynecology, psychiatry, radiation oncology, radiology, anesthesiology, and occupational medicine. Most surgical specialties require a five- to seven-year commitment.

The years of training and personal sacrifice should make you take a long, hard look at the medical profession. Although interesting and challenging, the sacrifice to yourself and your present or future family should be weighted heavily in your decision to choose medicine as a career.

"You move, seemingly not fast enough, to the head of the bed and a face from a horror movie stares up at you. Blood bubbles and froths out through the nose and mouth and oozes slowly down the cheeks to trickle onto the bed in streams like molten lava.

"'Suction!' You hear yourself speak in a voice half an octave above normal. An unseen hand places into one of yours a hissing plastic rod. With your hand, you reach down to open the bloody lips and pry apart the jaws to insert the vacuum tube and suck out the blood and vomitus so the patient can breathe. But the mouth . . . won't . . . open!"

FINANCING

The financial debt incurred as a result of selecting a medical career is often substantial. In addition to paying for four years of college, you will pay tuition costs of $2,500 to $30,000 a year for your medical training.

Although you will be compensated during your residency, the salary is low considering the loan payments you may be making. Most residents earn $20,000 to $30,000 per year. For this amount, the work load is staggering. It is fairly common for a resident to work a 120-hour work week on a regular basis. A surgeon summed up his residency training by stating, "I learned not to total up how many hours a week I worked. It was much easier to keep track of the hours I spent at home." Another commented, "If they would only pay us minimum wage I would be rich! Do you realize I earn less than $3.65 per hour?"

If your goal in life is wealth, there are much easier ways to attain it than through a medical career. While it is true most doctors make incomes ranging from $80,000 to $120,000 a year, many physicians accept the traditionally more challenging and interesting university-based academic hospital positions, which pay less. Since you will be 32 to 35 years old before you start earning a large salary and will have approximately $50,000 to $150,000 in debts, it may be much easier to attain wealth in a business career.

"A plastic collar wrapped around the patient's neck, placed in the field by the paramedics as protection against further injury to the neck, prevents opening the airway. 'Doctor, look at his lips!' one nurse shouts as she begins to cut away the patient's clothing, stiffened by drying blood and dirt. Through the sheen of red you see the lips are now a frightening shade of purple. Even as the second nurse removes the stethoscope from

her ears after taking a pulse and blood pressure reading and begins to
speak, you know what she will say, but you don't want to hear it.
  " 'We're losing him!'
  "You refrain from offering a silent prayer because there isn't time."

HELPING PEOPLE

The opportunity to help people is a major attraction to the medical profession. One has only to see the joy on the faces of a young patient and
his parents at discharge after recovery from what seemed to be a terminal
illness to appreciate the unique opportunity physicians have to affect
peoples' lives. Following the course of a comatose car accident victim
with multiple organ injuries from the emergency room to discharge, fully
recovered four weeks later gives the physician much satisfaction. Even
when a cure is not possible, a physician can find fulfillment in pallia-
tively treating a terminally ill cancer patient and enabling him to go home
and enjoy quality, albeit limited, time with his family and friends.

Caring for sick people is not glamorous. When people are sick they
usually exhibit their worst behavior. Illness transforms many people from
likable human beings to demanding tyrants. They are not happy to see
you because they do not feel well. If you cannot cure them quickly, their
frustration with the situation may lead to an unhappy patient-physician
relationship. The image of a physician as a knight in shining armor is
quickly tarnished by patients who cough on you, vomit on you, or worse!
The glamour of medicine fades quickly in the reality of a busy hospital.

  " 'Doctor, the pulse is weak at 40 and the blood pressure is 80/0.'
  "The first nurse has the upper clothes off—the patient suddenly be-
comes human. My God, she can't be more than 15!
  "The chest moves, but feebly, the muscles of respiration weakened by
the lack of air. She is breathing some, but not enough. A vicious cycle is
unfolding before your eyes. The resistance to air flowing into her lungs is
increased by the injuries to her nose and mouth. She needs more strength
to overcome this—but the harder she struggles to breathe, the weaker she
gets without air. Soon, she will stop breathing entirely. It seems like hours.
A minute and 27 seconds have passed."

Few of your patients will be the nice, little old lady who lives down
the street. Some of them, especially in the university or inner-city hospitals where you will probably train, will be indigent patients, most of whom
do not take good care of their health. They care as little for your help as
they do for themselves. These individuals are often jobless, homeless,

and without families. As a result, many of them have lost their personal dignity. Often they have chronic recurring diseases exacerbated by their lack of ability or desire to seek early medical care. The patients may be passive, may show you little respect, and will often disregard your medical advice. Yet you will spend many hours of your day and night treating these individuals. Caring for a patient who has lost a leg because of the arterial blockage caused by his smoking, and watching him sneak into a bathroom for a cigarette while the toes on the other foot turn blue from the same process, is to incur the frustration you will experience time and again as a healer.

"Why is her heartbeat so slow? If she is in shock from bleeding, it should be fast! Maybe she is bleeding into her head—that would cause bradycardia, but then her blood pressure should be high. But not if she is bleeding internally. The cardiac output is the product of the stroke volume multiplied by the heart rate with a value of 5 liters per minute in a normal 70-kilogram male at rest. A million useless facts, the end result of countless hours of study, suddenly crowd your mind—all except the one needed to save this girl's life."

IDEALS

The medical school experience will radically change your perception of life, death, suffering, and sacrifice. A number of interesting studies have been done on medical students and physicians. One study suggests that three experiences truly change a person's life: war, becoming a mother, and becoming a physician. Doctors have one of the highest suicide rates in the United States, second only to dentists. Another study analyzed professional student idealism. Medical students scored the highest in idealistic attitudes as freshmen compared to other professionals. However, by their senior year, they scored the lowest in idealism and highest in cynicism.

"'Doctor, what are you going to do?' asks the nurse, an edge of panic creeping into her voice.

"Her nose is broken, so you can't put a tube into her lungs through there. Even if her mouth opens, you won't be able to stretch out her neck enough to put in the tube. Amidst the noise of the emergency room and the jumble of thoughts racing through your head an idea takes hold and repeats itself incessantly . . . something you knew from the start but refused to acknowledge until now. I can't do that—I've never done it before! Even as you begin to speak, 'Get me a . . . '"

Medicine, for all its trials and tribulations, is a rewarding profession! Few physicians would select a different career if they had a choice to live their lives again. Yet, approaching medicine realistically is important. You must have an appreciation for what you are getting yourself into.

"The smooth neck is surprisingly free of blood; it resembles a stained wood log from the iodine disinfectant. One nurse stands holding the head between her hands to keep the neck from moving, the other across the patient ready to assist. With a tremble you attribute to high circulating levels of epinephrine, your left hand descends to the groove of bone at the base of the throat where previously nestled a heart-shaped pendant. Moving straight up the skin of the neck, your fingers feel the faint grooves of the trachea, followed by a small ridge—not unlike a speed-bump, you recall your instructor had said—the cricoid cartilage. Just above this is a soft depression, not larger than the tip of your finger. You repeat the process to confirm the landmark and though you wouldn't admit it, delay a bit to give somebody that knows what he's doing a chance to show up."

If you are undecided about a medical career, take time to experience the profession as much as possible. As a high school student or college freshman, try to find a volunteer or part-time position in a hospital. Be sure to experience the profession vicariously. The list at the end of the chapter includes books that hold both positive and negative views of a medical career. Take the time to read several books from both extremes. Do not let this chapter discourage you, but do take the time for an honest look at your motivations for selecting a medical career. Medicine is a hard road and a hard life. Most doctors believe it is worth it.

"You place your middle finger below the cricoid cartilage and the index finger above to stretch and fix the skin in place, leaving the depression unseen but marked by the finger's perimeter. Your right hand holds the handle of the scalpel correctly, as you were taught, with the butt of the handle nestled in the palm of your hand, the index finger resting above the stem of the blade and steadied by the grasp of the thumb and middle finger. You press down upon the skin and it parts, but only slightly. With more confidence you retrace the previous path, pushing through the skin, and are rewarded with a thin smile of blood. Taking but a second, you push the tip of your finger into the incision and feel the depression—the cricothyroid membrane. The nurse pats away the blood as you withdraw your finger. Using the front edge of the scalpel blade, you cut through the thin, tough membrane into the tracheal airway. Droplets of blood spew into the air like a geyser as the patient coughs reflexively. Dropping the

scalpel, you pick up the tracheostomy tube and with some difficulty force it into the opening. Quickly you remove the inner obturator, attach a ventilation unit, and rhythmically squeeze the black plastic bag, pumping pure oxygen into her lungs. Her lips are still blue, and, in your heart, you know you're too late."

Books You Should Read

Gordon, Noah. *The Death Committee*. Fawcett, 1969.

Gross, Martin L. *The Doctors*. Dell, 1967.

Illich, Ivan. *Medical Nemesis: The Expropriation of Health*. Pantheon, 1976.

Karp, Lawrence E., M.D. *The Hospital: The View From Bellevue*. Ace/Charter, 1979.

Laster, Leonard, ed. *Life After Medical School: Thirty-Two Doctors Describe How They Shaped Their Medical Careers*. W.W. Norton & Company, 1996.

Mendelsohn, Robert S., M.D. *Confessions of a Medical Heretic*. Warner Books, 1980.

Nolen, William A., M.D. *Making of a Surgeon*. Random House, 1970.

Seager, Stephen B., M.D. *Emergency*. Zebra Books, 1983.

Shem, Samuel, M.D. *The House of God*. Dell, 1981.

HIGH SCHOOL PREPARATION AND COLLEGE SELECTION

"Education is not the accumulation of knowledge, but the ability to find it."

Louis Nizer, J.D.

While attending high school, you can begin preparing yourself for a medical career. The approach taken will have a direct influence on your chances of becoming a physician. Now is the time to develop study habits that will help you do well in college and beyond. You should begin learning the good oral and written communication skills that are necessary in dealing with patients. A solid curriculum that will provide a foundation for future college courses is crucial. Selecting extracurricular activities that are enjoyable and emphasize the work ethic will develop your ability to survive medical training. Finally, it is time to analyze colleges, as a wise choice will improve your chances of gaining medical school admission.

EXPLORING MEDICINE AS A CAREER

As a high school or college student, it is difficult to know if medicine is the career for you. To make a realistic appraisal, you need to explore the medical profession in ways that will help you make an honest and planned career choice.

9

It is never too early to find a job in a hospital. Chapter 9 is devoted to helping you obtain such a position. As a high school student it may be better to start in a volunteer position to gain confidence, experience, and maturity working with people. Later, you may apply for one of the more exciting and demanding hospital jobs.

Working in a hospital may help you begin to understand what physicians do, but one important point should be emphasized. Even if you dislike the function you perform, such as EKG technician or phlebotomist, remember that your job in no way reflects what a physician actually does and experiences. For example, the sometimes boring and tedious job of drawing blood is a far cry from the demanding and intellectually challenging job of being a hospital pathologist. Your goal in doing any of these jobs is to observe and analyze. Keep your eyes and ears open to what doctors are doing, not to the limitations of your present hospital employment.

CLASSES

Excelling in college requires a strong foundation. You must take classes that will help you do well in college premedical courses. This means taking classes in biology, chemistry, physics, and mathematics. In addition, you should take courses that will develop your oral and written communication skills.

In your high school, you may have the opportunity to take college-level courses. This is a good idea if you use it as a testing ground. For example, taking a college-level inorganic chemistry course will enable you to determine your ability to handle college-level science courses. However, exercise caution, because the advanced placement class you take in high school may not actually involve college-level course work.

For example, if you take college-level Physics I in high school and arrive at college supposedly ready to take Physics II, you may be in for a shock when you find your knowledge base is not what it should be to tackle such a course. It may simply not be worth the risk. A grade of "B" or worse in a course that counts toward your science grade point average can jeopardize your future. However, if you start college with Physics I and do well because you took a similar course in high school, that good grade will contribute to your science grade point average. The same argument can apply to taking college-level inorganic chemistry, calculus, and biology courses. It is much better to repeat a course for an "A" than start at a higher level, which may result in less than "A" performance.

A similar consideration applies to CLEPping out of college-level course work. If you CLEP out of Inorganic Chemistry and start upper-division Organic Chemistry competing against sophomores and juniors, you may spoil your chances of doing "A" work in an important course. It would be much better to repeat and do well in inorganic chemistry and be fully prepared for organic chemistry.

COLLEGE SELECTION

Selecting a college will be one of the most difficult decisions you face. Much of the decision will be based on your personality. If you like large campuses, a major university may be the best choice. On the other hand, many students find a small college fulfills their needs. Either choice can provide the preparation you need for medical school.

Many bright students choose top competitive universities. Although these may be prestigious, they may or may not help you get into medical school. The old saying "It is easier to be a big fish in a small pond" is worth remembering. If you know that you are one of the gifted few who will do well wherever you attend college, then the most competitive school available can be an appropriate choice. However, if you are average or slightly above average, selecting a school that allows you to excel will be crucial to your future chances of being admitted to medical school.

College recruiters will cite high medical school acceptance rates to entice you to select their institution. Be cautious! For example, one school claims a 95 percent acceptance rate for their students applying to medical school. What they do not tell potential applicants is that their college has a medical school selection committee that prescreens applicants interested in applying to medical school. Only those individuals preselected by the "Medical School Committee" are given the necessary letter of recommendation to make acceptance into medical school a near certainty.

Another factor to consider is the percentage of premedical students who are "weeded out." One university claimed a 90 percent acceptance rate into medical school. Out of a freshman class of 1,600, 800 of whom initially declared themselves as premed, only 80 survived freshman and sophomore "weed-out" courses to become medical school applicants. In reality, the acceptance rate was less than 10 percent of the students initially interested in becoming physicians.

When evaluating your college choice, consider what percentage of the freshman class are premeds. This statistic will give you a strong indication of how competitive the school will be. If you are careful in your selection of a college, this may work to your advantage. For example, a small state school that is not well known as a premedical school may have less competition and provide better chances of surviving the four years of premedical course work. Perhaps only five to ten graduates are accepted into medical school each year from a student body of 1,000. If there are only 20 premed freshman a year, and 15 survive to apply to medical school, with 10 accepted, the actual odds of getting into medical school are much better than the college previously discussed, which advertised a 90 percent acceptance rate!

An important factor to consider in selecting a college is to choose a state where it is less difficult to get into medical school. If you are from California, New York, or any of the other heavily populated states, now may be the time to establish residency in a state where the number of applicants applying to medical school is much smaller. Future chapters address methods to determine which states fall into this category. Although you may eventually return to California, it is much easier to find a spot in a California residency program than it is to find a medical school position.

Some colleges are affiliated with medical schools. Often these schools will show a degree of favoritism toward their undergraduates in selecting their medical school class. Schools prone to doing this will often show similar favoritism toward applicants who have had previous family members attend their institution. These factors must be considered on an individual basis.

In selecting your undergraduate institution, take the time to list all the advantages and disadvantages of each school you are considering. Try to consider as many factors as possible in making your decision. Even though you may want to please your parents by selecting their alma mater, keep in mind the importance of choosing a school that will enhance your medical school admission chances.

HIGH SCHOOL PERFORMANCE AND COLLEGE ENTRANCE EXAMS

Believe it or not, high school performance has little to do with your ability to do well in college. You will be amazed at the number of valedictorian high school graduates who fail to continue their exceptional performance at the college level.

There are many reasons for performance to change dramatically as a high school student enters college. Some high school students were pushed by parents to study all the time, and when they go away to college they find partying is much easier than studying. Other students used their maximum abilities to do well at the high school level and now, as they reach a higher level of competition at college, do not have the reserve to continue to succeed. Still others go from average to excellent performance when they reach college. For example, some students who were in multiple activities in high school, which interfered with their study time and focus, now have a new level of dedication to their studies as college students. Some excel in college because it allows them to take more classes that interest them. A few students found high school too easy and consequently did not even try. In college they are faced with tough courses and rise to the occasion. Whatever the reason, being a star in high school will not guarantee future success. College is a whole new ball game requiring a greater level of determination and skills to do well.

Most high school counselors will use ACT and SAT scores to measure your ability to succeed in college. Although test scores determine scholarships and perhaps where you go to college, they have little influence on your chances of acceptance into medical school. Few medical schools ask for your college entrance exam scores on their application. Medical school admissions tests are radically different from college entrance exams. Hard work and perseverance in college science courses will play a much greater role in how well you do on medical school entrance exams. The average student accepted into medical school has only a slightly better score than the national average of college student ACT and SAT scores.

COMBINED DEGREE PROGRAMS

Several colleges offer a combined degree program. They provide students with an opportunity to be selected for medical school based on their high school performance. Most offer B.S.-M.D. degrees to individuals completing their programs. Advantages of these programs include a near guarantee of being accepted into medical school and in a possibly shorter time span (usually six years versus the traditional eight years to complete the program). In addition, the shorter time in some instances can reduce the student's overall cost of completing a medical education. Requirements of students usually include a minimum grade point average and Medical College Admission Test score.

There are disadvantages to a combined degree program. One major disadvantage is that you may feel locked into a medical career before having had sufficient time to consider other career choices. A second disadvantage, especially for gifted students, is that you may be locked into attending a medical school that is not equal to your abilities. A third problem is that your college program may be narrowed to such a degree that you do not have the time to take nonscience courses. Missing out on a strong humanities background can be detrimental to your ability to communicate with and understand your future patients. Finally, a few schools make it exceedingly difficult to complete the program. The acceptance rate of individuals completing the program should be carefully weighed.

When selecting a combined degree program, seek out the opinions of students already in the program. In addition, make sure the program has a mechanism for your completing college should you decide to apply to another medical school or seek a different career.

Selecting a career as a physician requires thought. Early preparation for the long and arduous road you will face is crucial. As a high school student, begin to build a foundation. It is important that you learn the basics of science, math, writing, and reading, develop oral communication skills, and select a college that allows you to perform to the best of your abilities, thus enhancing your chances of gaining admission to medical school.

C H A P T E R   3

COLLEGE PROFESSORS / ADVISORS

"**The mediocre teacher tells. The good teacher explains. The superior teacher demonstrates. The great teacher inspires.**"

William Arthur Ward

Highly motivated, stimulating, brilliant college professors are the ideal. Unfortunately, not all college professors meet these high standards. The realities about college professors must be faced. Some instructors, brilliant in their subject matter, lack basic teaching skills. Understanding the motivations of professors can help you understand and prevent problems that may arise in your college education.

COLLEGE PROFESSORS

Education

College professors often lack the educational training to help them become great teachers. Most of the really talented instructors simply have the personality and natural ability to teach well.

Why are some college instructors poor teachers? The answer to this question is best considered by way of example. Take the average chemistry professor, just out of graduate school. He is assigned to teach an introductory inorganic chemistry course. As a college student he majored in chemistry and took the same basic courses you are in, progressing through the ranks of advanced chemistry course work. Later, he continued his pursuit of chemistry with advanced undergraduate work in organic, analytical, and physical chemistry. Never, however, in his final years of college chemistry did he take further work in the fundamental principles of inorganic chemistry. After graduating from college, he began a six- to seven-year study of a specialized field of chemistry to earn his master's degree and doctorate. This entailed advanced courses in highly specialized areas culminating in a long and arduous research thesis on a specific topic. This topic addressed one question about an obscure point in his specialized area of chemistry, most probably dealing with a single aspect of complex chemical principles.

This individual is hired to teach an inorganic chemistry course at the college you are attending. He does have expertise in his own research area of chemistry. However, he has a limited knowledge of the vast array of material presented in an inorganic chemistry course. Like his students, he must read the text and review the "general principles" to present to the class. Soon, he may become disinterested and bored with presenting general principles to students year after year.

Teaching Experience

Many college professors are not prepared to teach because they have limited training in how to give lectures, write exams, prepare notes, or use audiovisual aids. In short, they lack training in the fine art of conveying information at the introductory level. Some professors are nervous talking to a class of 400 freshman. The average college professor has not had the benefit of four years of teaching-method courses that high school instructors are required to complete. As a consequence, they often lack the knowledge, and sometimes ability, to give good lectures.

Teaching Incentive

At some institutions, instructors have little or no incentive to make teaching a high priority. Young faculty members' primary goal is to publish, as this strongly influences their chances of becoming tenured and making full professor. Their own research is much more important to them than spending time preparing a well-organized lecture. Many selected academic careers not for love of teaching, but for love of research, and the time they spend teaching stands in the way of their own goals.

Grades

Any college senior, after years of experience, will tell you the secret of doing well in college is not what courses you take but whom you take them with. You will be surprised the first time a college professor tells you a specific subject will not be on an exam and you find not one, but several, questions on that very topic. You will be even more amazed at the college professor who writes with one hand and erases with the other, making it impossible for you to take class notes. Worse are instructors whose lectures are so nonspecific, disjointed, and convoluted that you have no idea what is important, and yet whose exams are masterpieces of small bits of data that seemingly fail to appear anywhere in your notes or textbook. Eventually, you find the answer to the question buried in the footnote of the textbook chapter you were told to "skim briefly." Some examinations will make even the best-prepared students wonder if they were even given the correct test.

Why are many college exams impossible? Because teachers must "weed you out." Let's face it: Most college-level material makes sense to individuals of average intelligence. If prepared, even the nongifted should be able to comprehend most college courses. Unfortunately, only a small percent of students are allowed to do well in college, especially in science courses, so that only the best and brightest will have grades that let them seek admission to medical school. Not everyone can be a doctor, so college instructors must maintain tests at a level of difficulty that selects only the top students. Since the material in most classes is relatively straightforward, and premedical students are highly motivated to learn the material, professors are forced to use every means available to make challenging exams. The easiest way to do this is to use tools such as deceit, trick questions, lack of organization, and an insufficient amount of time to complete exams. All of these test tactics make preparation difficult and exceedingly frustrating.

PREMEDS—THE WORST KIND OF STUDENTS

Premeds are in a very precarious position. Many college instructors, particularly science instructors, dislike premeds! Why? (1) You are probably not taking chemistry because you have an honest desire to learn chemistry, but because you need it to get into medical school; and (2) you are very grade conscious and will take every opportunity to increase your scores (such as by constantly badgering your instructors for extra points).

This attitude on your part is irritating to your professors. After all, they have dedicated their lives to science and have little appreciation for your need to learn only a fraction of their field.

These generalizations should not destroy your faith in your college education, because there will be many teachers who will inspire you to learn, work, and study to be the best student you can be. At any college, many people teach because they enjoy teaching and are excellent instructors. The problem is, early in your college career you probably have no idea who those instructors are or where to find them. Until you know which instructors to look for, you must develop a strategy to overcome or avoid the less-than-ideal teachers you face. This will eventually come with time and experience. However, time and experience are something for which the premed who must do well cannot wait. In future chapters, a strategy to succeed, in spite of adversity, will be fully developed.

COLLEGE ADVISORS

"Good advice is not cheap!" There is a big difference in the quality of premedical advisors. At some institutions, a talented, well-trained premedical advisor is available. Unfortunately, at many large undergraduate institutions, the number of freshman premed students leads to a big demand for premedical advisors. Often the individuals who fill this role are college professors with minimal counseling knowledge.

Here is an example of the danger of bad premedical advice. At one college a new premedical advisor's "training" consisted of a handout describing what classes were required to apply to medical school. With this in hand, he advised several freshman premeds to take Inorganic Chemistry I, General Biology I, General Physics I, English, and Calculus I as first-semester freshmen. The disaster a classmate experienced as a result of this advice led to three-and-a-half years of catch-up to overcome the 2.0 GPA he received.

Qualities to look for in a premedical advisor are experience and understanding. An advisor lacking the expertise to help you plan a reasonable freshman schedule is less than adequate. If your college assigns advisors and yours is questionable, look for a new one. Upperclassmen can often suggest an advisor who can meet your premedical needs. A good advisor should help you evaluate your strengths and weaknesses and assist you in forming a reasonable academic schedule. He or she should be someone to whom you can relate. Remember, in three years you may need to approach this individual for a letter of recommendation.

Finding someone who is not only an advisor but also a friend should be one of your highest priorities.

When you meet with your advisor, be prepared to ask what course options you have as a freshman. Be ready to admit your strengths and weaknesses so that he or she can assist you in making up any deficits you have. If disaster should strike, such as a bad grade, ask how the effects can be minimized. Remember, advisors judge you when they meet with you; do not be afraid and do not try to manipulate them—your advisor will see through it. Listen to what your advisor says, and be sure to thank him or her for suggestions and advice.

A well-informed advisor should have access to two publications that may help as you progress through your premedical training. One is *The Advisor*, a newsletter for advisors tailored to premedical students. The other is the *Journal of Medical Education*, which provides up-to-date information on medical college admissions scores, grade point averages, financial information, and a variety of other topics useful in making premedical decisions.

As a freshman, you are at a very dangerous point in your career. You are faced with the possibility of poor instruction and poor advice. Often the winds of fate are allowed to determine your ultimate success in your quest to get into medical school. This may have very little to do with your actual ability, motivation, or desire. So if you want to get into medical school, the sooner you learn to control your destiny with regard to instructors and advisors, the better your chances of success!

CHAPTER 4

FRESHMAN CLASSES

**"I have learned not to be frightened by discourage-
ment. I've come to believe that profound hopeless-
ness is often a necessary catharsis. Only when you
can accept the facts of what didn't work can you go
on to find what does."**

Rev. Leonard L. Smalls

When will you realize how tough it is to get into medical school? Too
often, the dream of an easy ticket evaporates after the first inorganic chemistry exam. After looking at your test score, you realize that if you get 95
on the next four exams, you might get a "B" in the class.

In high school it was easy for students to do well, because the competition was not as keen. College is a new ball game. Chemistry class may
be composed of 199 students who did as well as you did in high school
chemistry. Most of them have the same goal that you do: They want to be
doctors and are determined to let nothing stand in their way.

The solution: *Do not be overconfident!* Most freshmen begin by taking too difficult a class load. Freshman courses are sometimes the most
challenging in your college career. Not only are you inexperienced in
meeting the demands of college course work, but these courses tend to be
"weed-out classes" designed to be difficult.

What can you do about it?

PLAN AHEAD

Know your abilities. Be aware that college life, especially the first semester, offers many distractions. You will be away from home for the first time and responsible for learning a large volume of material; classes will be more competitive; and most important, you will not yet know the system. However, by following some guidelines you can increase your chances of having a successful freshman year.

Number one: Use the class "drop" system to your advantage. There are several drop deadlines. Know the drop date that will enable you to withdraw from a class without putting a withdraw (W) or withdraw failing (WF) on your transcript. This deadline is usually two to three weeks into the semester. There is also a second drop date, the one the school commonly "advertises," which is usually six to eight weeks into the semester. On occasion, especially during freshman year, you may use this second deadline, which permanently records a "W" on your transcript. This is undesirable, but one "W" is far better than a "C" grade or worse!

Now that you know that dropping a class is a possibility, plan your schedule with dropping in mind. You will soon learn that at least two-thirds of your professors will be good teachers. Sign up for eighteen hours knowing that you may be dropping at least one and possibly two classes. Try to do it before the second transcript deadline, but drop anytime if you must. After your freshman year you will know who the good teachers are, will have developed better study habits, and will know the system, reducing your need to drop a class. As a freshman, you want to look your best, and 12 or 15 hours of "A" and one "W" looks far better than a "C" in any class!

Number two: Plan an easy schedule. As a freshman, you do not know which classes are easy and which are difficult. Most freshman science and required classes are difficult. This is because many freshmen are taking the classes, making competition fierce. In addition, instructors generally dislike teaching freshman classes for reasons previously discussed. Often graduate assistants, students themselves, teach and grade these classes.

Graduate students, as a rule, dislike premeds, and for good reason: (1) You do not have the same level of interest in the materials that they do, (2) most graduate students competed against premeds at some point in their career and may have done poorly in a class because "some premed gunner" destroyed the curve, and (3) you are more concerned about getting an "A" in the class than in appreciating the material.

There are solutions to your scheduling problem as a freshman. First, find less difficult classes. Old standbys include classes in anthropology, physical education, sociology, and psychology. Remember, there is a degree of variance between institutions, so check out a course ahead of time. Even if the class does not fulfill a core requirement, still take it, because you can always make up a core requirement at a later date. At this point, your goal is to get past the freshman year with a reasonable grade point average.

Second, upperclassmen are another good source of class information, so talk to as many as possible. Ask them which classes are good and who are the best teachers. Find out the degree of difficulty of each class.

Third, required humanities classes are often difficult. It is in your best interest to find humanities classes that will interfere least with the study time needed to do well in introductory science classes.

Fourth, if your science skills are weak, think seriously about not taking more than one science class per semester of your freshman year, and this should be your best science subject. You need at least a "B" if you want to get into medical school, and 80 percent of your effort will probably be channeled in this direction. This is why you are signing up for other "easy" classes—because science classes must be your primary concern.

Fifth, most medical schools require calculus. Do not take this your freshman year unless you had two semesters of college-level calculus in high school, and never sign up for advanced placement in calculus. As a freshman, you will compete against students from high schools where two to three semesters of calculus were taught. The students you are competing against in college may be repeating calculus and will have a distinct advantage. It is preferable to repeat an advanced algebra class the first semester and start Calculus I in the off semester, when you are competing against people with weaker or similar academic backgrounds. Plus, you need the time for your science class, and having to complete calculus homework will not make your job any easier! Medical schools do not look at your high school transcripts, so if repeating Advanced Algebra or Calculus I is an easy "A" in your freshman year, go for it!

Sixth, take the time to see potential instructors prior to registration. Most college professors will be happy to discuss their course and give you an idea whether your background is sufficient to excel in the class.

Finally, know your strengths and weaknesses. How quick are you to grasp a new math, science, English, or historical concept? Some people are good at quantitative skills, such as physics and math, and others at qualitative skills, such as reading and writing. Whatever the case, as a freshman, take classes that emphasize your strengths. For example, avoid freshman history if it is not one of your best subjects. If you like biology, take it rather than chemistry or physics. Put off dealing with your weaknesses until your sophomore year, when you have a better grasp of your abilities and can select the best instructors.

So what should a freshman schedule look like?

At Registration	
Chemistry, Physics, or Biology	3 hours
Lab	1 hour
Algebra or Calculus I	3 hours
Physical Education	1 hour
Major, if known	3 hours
Core Requirement A	3 hours
Core Requirement B	3 hours
Total	17 hours

Before the first drop deadline (No "W"!), drop a class if you are doing poorly. Your schedule should now look something like this:

At First Drop Deadline	
Chemistry, Physics, or Biology	3 hours
Lab	1 hour
Algebra or Calculus	3 hours
Physical Education	1 hour
Major	3 hours
Core Requirement A or B	3 hours
Total	14 hours

At the second drop deadline, consider dropping one more class if you have a poor shot at an "A," or at least a "B." If you had an unsalvageable disaster on a first exam, dropping should be strongly considered. You will try to end up with 11 to 14 hours of "A" and no more than one "W," which, if you "wake up" by second semester, will not happen again. If you have to drop the science class, continue to show up for class and take practice copies of the exams. You must be ready to get an "A" when you pick this class up again next semester. As it will now be in the off semester, you may find the competition and class size reduced, improving your chances for success. The second semester of the two-semester science sequence will have to be completed during the summer, but you will have fared much better and avoided what might have been an insurmountable task. Remember, if you want to get into medical school, plan ahead; know what to take, when to take it, and when to drop; and be very careful in selecting your first-semester classes.

CHAPTER 5

MAJOR SELECTION

"Change and Growth take place when a person has
risked himself and dares to become involved with
experimenting with his own life."

Herbert Otto

It is a well-kept secret that you can major in anything you want and get
into medical school! Most students take the traditional biology, chemistry, or physics route, but in reality any major is acceptable. Freshman
often select a science major thinking it will help them get into medical
school or make medical school easier. They are probably wrong on both
accounts.

SCIENCE MAJORS

Majoring in science is usually more difficult than majoring in other subjects, because you are competing with a greater proportion of premeds.
For example, if you apply to medical school with a biology major, you
are automatically in a large pool of biology major applicants. To succeed
from this position requires an outstanding performance. You had better
be one of the best swimmers in the pool if you hope to get into medical
school.

The argument is often made that being a science major will help in
medical school. In general, this is not true. There are only a few instances
where physics principles are used in medicine, and these are learned
in introductory physics courses. The only chemistry used in medicine
beyond a few principles from inorganic and organic chemistry is taught

in biochemistry. Completing four years of chemistry for one biochemistry course is unnecessary, especially since the only prerequisites for biochemistry are freshman-level biology and inorganic and organic chemistry.

Surprisingly, biology majors do not always have an advantage in medical school. At most undergraduate schools, they are required to take several courses in plant biology and ecology. Of the animal science classes taken, few will be in human biology. The human biology classes that are offered are open to all students and often require only freshman biology as a prerequisite.

One major value of any science course is the memorization skills learned. This is important! However, these skills can be acquired in select classes that will help you in medical school, such as biochemistry, histology, embryology, genetics, and physiology. Because these classes can be taken after meeting freshman biology and chemistry prerequisites, you need not be a science major to benefit from taking these upper-division courses. However, if you see an interesting science course taught by an instructor you like, do not hesitate to take it, even if it does not cover a medical school topic, as it will still improve your memorization skills.

If you really like biology, chemistry, or physics, do not be afraid to select a science major in a subject area you enjoy, but realize the benefits and risks. Physics is a good major if it is a subject you can grasp and master with a minimum of work. However, it requires a significant number of support classes. For example, majors in physics or chemistry may require you to take 30 hours of physics or chemistry classes and Calculus I through Calculus III, Differential Equations, and Statistics. This limits free time to take other, biologically based science courses for a well-rounded science background and biology classes that will help you in medical school. It also means you will take four or five difficult science classes along with your premedical science requirements.

SELECTING A MAJOR

So which major should you choose? Consider a different major from what most other premeds select. A major with a low number of total hour requirements is preferable. For example, an English major may require as little as 24 course hours. This allows free time to take science classes. It also places you in a competitive position for top grades in introductory-level science classes. While the science majors are overwhelmed, preparing themselves for three to five science classes, you are making preparations for only one or two and can give each class your best effort. Being a nonscience major, you will be able to pick and choose the extra science courses that interest you rather than being forced to take a science course to complete your major.

In selecting a major, choose an area you enjoy. You probably will perform better if you major in something you find really interesting. If it is a major outside the traditional premed pool and you get to know one or two instructors well, you are more apt to obtain outstanding letters of recommendation, since your instructors are not comparing you with the large number of science major premeds. Another advantage is that when you do take an extra science class, you can select the very best instructors. For example, if histology is taught by an outstanding instructor, take it; if the embryology class is bad, skip it. This is a luxury your science major friends may not have. You may also take the same excellent science instructor several times, which should make getting a science letter of recommendation much easier.

Nearly any major is acceptable, though a few are better than others. Speech, English, communications, and journalism are excellent, because they teach oral and written communication skills that are essential in medicine. A language major is an excellent choice if you have a talent for picking up languages, especially since it teaches you to memorize. The average freshman medical student learns 10,000 new words his or her first year, and the ability to learn a new vocabulary will be very helpful. Anthropology and psychobiology tend to be excellent majors, although they require a few extra courses in peripheral fields. History and political science majors are a fair choice, although they do not give you much cushion if you change your career plans. An economics major is unusual, but you must get the degree outside a business school to avoid a number of required support courses. This degree also offers an alternative if your medical school plans fail to materialize.

Business majors are acceptable, but most business degrees require peripheral course work. For example, a management major would be helpful in medicine; however, this would require introductory courses in accounting, economics, finance, marketing, statistics, and computers. A math major is fine if you are adept at math. In general, the major does not require a significant amount of peripheral course work. Math courses also count toward your science grade point average, which is a bonus when you prepare your medical school application.

One approach to selecting a major is to obtain a copy of your school's handbook. It lists majors and their requirements for graduation. Look for a major that interests you, but also consider the time factor. You must have free time for your science classes. Once you have found two or three possible majors, go to those departments and look for upperclassmen. Ask pertinent questions, such as "Do you like this major? How good are the instructors? Who are the good instructors? Is it a difficult major?" Armed with this information, choose a class sometime during your freshman year and see if the major agrees with you.

A thought to keep in mind when you do select a major is whether you can do something else with it if you decide not to go to medical school. Also, consider your hobbies and interests when selecting a major. If art is your hobby, why not spend four years of your life developing that interest for a later time when you can enjoy it.

One of the most valuable books to examine before selecting a major is *Medical School Admission Requirements,* sponsored by the Association of American Medical Colleges. It provides an accurate analysis of the percent of acceptance rates for most college majors. Although acceptance rates vary from year to year, physical science tends to score the highest acceptance rates, with majors in biomedical engineering, chemical engineering, and electrical engineering leading the group. Surprisingly, the traditional premedical biological science majors of biology, microbiology, zoology, and physiology carry much lower acceptance rates.

Of the nonscience majors, economics, anthropology, English, history, psychobiology, and foreign languages came out on top. Lower acceptance rates were noted in sociology and psychology.

Overall, physical science majors have an above-average acceptance rate, nonscience majors tend to be slightly lower, and biological science majors, surprisingly, have the lowest average acceptance rate. Double nonscience majors tend to do slightly better than double science majors. Premedicine majors tend to fare only slightly better than biological science majors. Students able to handle a variety of subjects do well, as interdisciplinary study majors tend to have a very high acceptance rate.

As the trends suggest, selecting a nontraditional major may be an important consideration for gaining acceptance into a medical school. If you are not accepted or your career plans change, you can always stay in college a fifth year and pursue a more practical course. Keep in mind that if you want to go to medical school, an unusual interesting major you like may increase your odds of gaining medical school acceptance!

INFORMATION SOURCES

Medical education issue, *Journal of the American Medical Association.* Vol. 256, No. 12, September 1986.

Medical School Admission Requirements. 1998. Association of American Medical Colleges, 2450 N Street N.W., Washington, D.C. 20037-1127.

CHAPTER 6

CORE REQUIREMENTS

"Life freed from all responsibility, or from ordinary
hardships retains little to urge man on to accomplishment."

Frederick E. Jackson, M.D.

Almost every college in the United States has courses termed "core requirements." Often they are introductory courses in art, math, history,
philosophy, speech, English, political science, psychology, economics,
sociology, computer science, theology, and sociology. They are designed
to provide a "well-rounded" education. In the ideal setting, they can be
one of the highlights of college. They can help you acquire new interests
outside your primary field of study, attain important qualitative skills and
social awareness, and appreciate and understand the broader scope of
human endeavor. Looking back on college, many graduates wish that
they had taken more of these courses and fewer classes directly pertinent
to their career goals.

Unfortunately, core requirements often do not live up to these high
ideals. In fact, they may turn out to be some of the worst courses of your
college career. Because they are basic courses, core requirements are often taught by graduate students or young, inexperienced professors. Since
every freshman is in one or more of these classes, the competition can be
intense.

Due to large class size, instructors in core courses are forced to take
what should be a straightforward course and make it exceedingly
difficult. Grading is usually tougher in these classes because of the large

number of students competing for a finite number of "A's." Adding to the difficulty is that as a freshman you are ill prepared to compete in these classes, especially since 20 to 30 percent of the class may be upperclassmen.

Fortunately, there are alternatives, such as saving core courses for the junior or senior year or taking them on a pass/fail basis. This eliminates the pressure of taking a difficult core course as a freshman. In addition, after the first two to three semesters of college you will be aware of which courses and instructors are of the highest quality. You will then be able to select the best core requirements for your sophomore and junior years. The poor or challenging courses can be taken in the senior year, when they will not appear on your application for medical school.

Admittedly, you will need to take one to two core requirements each semester of the freshman year. Your best strategy is to talk to upperclass-men *before* registration and find out about easy core classes. Be prepared to drop one core requirement by taking at least one extra class. If circum-stances force you to drop two core requirements, you can usually take an extra course during the three-week summer pre-session, which starts just after the second semester. Summer sessions often have fewer students, and instructors thus tend to grade more according to the effort the student displays. Also, since you will be taking just one course, you can concen-trate your efforts on doing well.

Most students take core requirements on blind faith, thinking that since they are "requirements" they do not demand careful preevaluation. This is the wrong attitude. For example, medical school selection committees will not know that you picked a core history requirement in Central Ameri-can history over American history because Central American history was more interesting to you, well taught, and fairly graded. However, if you unwisely chose a poor American history course and received a "C," they will be aware only of your poor performance. Core requirements may prove to be the most interesting courses in your college training, but they are one more obstacle to overcome!

SCIENCE GRADE MAINTENANCE

"The toughest thing about success is that you've got to keep on being a success."

Irving Berlin

Maintaining grades has been discussed at length: Learning to recognize borderline instructors, selecting the right courses, and delaying difficult classes until your senior year are all strategies for maintaining your grades. Some difficult courses, however, will have to be included in your schedule fairly early on, even though this violates the basic strategy discussed. These courses are usually introductory courses in inorganic and organic chemistry, biology, physics, statistics, and calculus, all of which are required for entry into medical school. They also constitute the prerequisites for later, more advanced courses that may be called for in your medical school application, and for that reason will have to be taken earlier than you might prefer.

FRESHMAN YEAR

Few freshmen realize that when these six science classes are completed, all the requirements for most medical schools have been met. Any other science classes taken will simply be to raise your science grade point average, make medical school easier, or enjoy the subject or teacher.

Raising your science grade point average is a consideration, but it is not a good reason to take a science class! If you did not do well in your basic science classes, there is no guarantee you will suddenly do well in the advanced courses. However, do not despair. Some people have difficulty adjusting to their first science courses and overcome these problems in the more advanced courses.

The best approach to meeting your premedical required courses is to do your best the first time. Of course, this is easier said than done, but there are a number of things you can do to help. The first is to spread the required science courses out. As previously described, one possible schedule is as follows:

First Semester

Inorganic I	4 hours
Algebra	3 hours
Physical Education	1 hour
Easy class	3 hours
Major, if known	3 hours
Core Requirement	3 hours
(Be prepared to drop 3 to 6 hours)	

Second Semester

Inorganic Chemistry II	4 hours
Calculus I	3 hours
Easy class	3 hours
Major	3 hours
Core Requirement	3 hours
Core Requirement	3 hours
(Be prepared to drop 3 hours; you should be wise enough at this point to make one bad choice, not two!)	
Pre-session	Make up dropped class
Summer School	Varies with first-year performance

Normally you can relax the summer following the freshman year. If you had to drop inorganic chemistry, you are obligated to retake this class during the summer months. The only reasonable pretext for dropping inorganic chemistry is a grade of "C" or less. Most medical school committees realize students are prepared for inorganic chemistry at different levels depending on their high school background and accept a "B." They do, however, frown on grades lower than an "A" in organic chemistry, which is in the sophomore curriculum. The solution is to obtain an "A" in this course.

There is only one way to do this. You must be prepared for organic! If you have a great deal of self-motivation, you can spend several hours a day reading an organic chemistry text during the summer. Another method, and perhaps the best, is to audit a summer-school organic chemistry class at an institution other than your own college. To audit a course, most schools will allow you to pay a reduced fee or ask the instructor's permission to sit in on the class at no charge. You may have to try several large state schools to find one that will allow you to do this, but in the greater scheme of things, the sacrifice is worth it. You may balk at the idea of spending your summer months sitting in an organic class, but organic is the course that makes or breaks many a premedical student's career, and it must be your priority to see that it is an obstacle you overcome.

SOPHOMORE YEAR

This is the year that decides whether you are medical school material, so you need to be very selective about the major and core classes you choose. Biology and organic together are challenge enough for any student. This year should consist of the lightest class load you can find outside of your science course work.

First Semester	
Biology I	4 hours
Organic I	4 hours
Major	3 hours
Core Requirement	3 hours
Core or Major	3 hours
Physical Education	1 hour

Second Semester	
Biology II	4 hours
Organic II	4 hours
Major	3 hours
Core Requirement	3 hours
Core or Major	3 hours
Physical Education	1 hour
Presession	Make up 3 hours of requirements if you were forced to drop any courses or if you want to lighten your semester schedule

JUNIOR YEAR

You may want to pick up one extra biology course each semester, especially if you did not "ace" both semesters of general biology. If you had an "A" both semesters, it may be better to leave well enough alone until the senior year. However, if one grade was lower than an "A," you are obliged to find an upper-biology course to demonstrate your ability in biology. Any biology class will do, but pick one that interests you and is taught by a good professor. You should consider a course in which you can excel, keeping in mind an "A" is imperative! One of your biology instructors will be writing you a letter of recommendation, so choose the instructor to whom you can best relate and get to know him or her.

First Semester	
Physics I	4 hours
Optional Biology	4 hours
Major	3 hours
Major	3 hours
Core Requirement	3 hours
Physical Education	1 hour

Second Semester	
Physics II	4 hours
Optional Biology	4 hours
Major	3 hours
Major	3 hours
Core Requirement	3 hours
Physical Education	1 hour
Summer	Study for the MCAT!

SENIOR YEAR

By now you are a seasoned college student and ready for those challenging classes you bypassed. Now is your opportunity to take a few courses to help make medical school a little easier. You should consider taking courses offered in human anatomy, histology, physiology, biochemistry, microbiology, embryology, or genetics. Although these upper-division biology classes are not necessary, they will sharpen your memorization skills and make the freshman year of medical school less stressful. The grades you receive in these classes do not appear on your application to medical school, so you can lighten up and take them for sheer enjoyment. This is also a good opportunity to complete undesirable core requirements and get tough major classes out of the way. Some of these may be taken pass/fail if you are concerned about destroying your grade point average.

First Semester	
Major	3 hours
Major or Core Requirement	3 hours
Core Requirement	3 hours
Histology	4 hours
Genetics	4 hours

Second Semester	
Major	3 Hours
Major or Core Requirement	3 hours
Biochemistry	4 hours
Human Anatomy	4 hours

The suggested scheduling is by no means the only way to arrange your college curriculum. You may find it necessary to take summer school classes to improve your science grades. You may also take more "major" classes than "core" classes earlier if you find the former easier. You must, above all, keep in mind your primary objective, which is to *maximize* your grade point average in the freshman, sophomore, and junior years. Overall, a science GPA of approximately 3.5 should make you a competitive applicant for most medical schools. If your science GPA is lower than this, you need to consider extra science course work. Plan science courses carefully. Save nonscience classes that will give you serious problems for your senior year, when the grades received will not have an effect on your chances of getting into medical school. Keep in mind, summer preparation may be the key to your success!

CHAPTER 8

STUDY HABITS

**"I know of no more encouraging fact than the
unquestionable ability of a man to elevate his life by
a conscious endeavor."**

Henry David Thoreau

Without a doubt, study skills lead the list of abilities necessary for success in both college and medical school. Good study habits demand more than cramming and pulling an "all-nighter" before a big test. Doing well in school requires an understanding of the material presented and an ability to recognize the intangible elements unique to every class. These intangibles make a difference in your final grade. The goal is to recognize and use these intangible elements to your advantage.

CLASS MATERIALS

One of the first things to do when starting a new class is to determine the study materials required. Before you run to the bookstore and buy the $85.00 textbook listed in the course catalog, contact an upperclassman who has already taken the course to determine whether the investment is necessary. Quite often instructors list a required text because it is department policy, then ignore the text and teach (and test) from their notes. If notes are important for the class, obtain a copy from an upperclassman. This gives you an extra set of notes to compare to your own. In addition, instructors often accidentally leave out key facts that may show up on exams. Last year's notes may help fill these important gaps! If you decide to purchase a text for a class, look around for used copies, as the purchase of a used text can save you 50 to 75 percent.

A common question raised by undergraduates at the beginning of every class is how important the old tests are. Old tests can be crucial. Certainly this is a question to ask the experienced upperclassmen. Obtain copies of these tests if indicated. In general, the best way to use them is to wait until you have gone over the material completely. In this way you will not only better prepare yourself for the upcoming test, but will enhance your understanding and appreciation of the material.

CLASS ANALYSIS

After you have the appropriate class materials, your next step is to classify each class as objective or subjective. Essentially, all college classes are on a continuum that can be described as subjective on one end and objective on the other. Subjective classes, such as philosophy and theology, rely more on interpretation and expansion of broad general principles than on the mastery (and memorization) of numerous facts and figures that are more indicative of an objective class, such as general chemistry, general biology, or calculus. Some classes, such as history and psychology, are a mixture of these two types. Making this distinction will be crucial in determining your game plan for approaching each class.

Subjective classes require memorization of a few facts and ideas, but certainly the emphasis is on development and extrapolation of these concepts. In most cases, testing in these classes will involve essay-type questions. It is important to gear your study for this format on three levels. Level one, the highest, involves understanding the basic concepts presented in class and using them as the framework on which to build an essay answer. For instance, if the topic covered concerns Marx and Engel's communist theories, then a basic understanding of the concepts is mandatory. The second level is gaining an appreciation for your professor's ideas on these basic concepts. If your professor is a Marxist, it would be to your advantage to structure your answers to his or her test questions appropriately. Finally, the third level involves your own creative ideas. Most teachers enjoy reading their student's appraisal of basic material as long as it is well presented. But be careful and always remember the old saying that "A person's favorite voice (and ideas) are still his own." In other words, express your opinion, but be careful not to contradict blatantly either the basic material or your professor's opinion of it.

Objective classes require an entirely different study technique. The key here is twofold: Get *all* the material that could possibly be on the test, and *learn* all the material that could be on the test. The most crucial thing to be done in this type of class is to analyze carefully materials needed, such as class notes, old tests, and texts, and go over them as many times as possible. Several scientific studies have shown that the greatest amount of learning takes place during the second and third time through material. So the golden rule in these classes is to *get it and go through it* until you know it.

TIME FRAME

One of the toughest questions to answer about college classes is how much one has to study to do well. In general, extremes are not the best way to go. Examples of this are studying 24 hours a day at the expense of hobbies, social activities, and exercise or postponing study until the week before the exam and then cramming and pulling all-nighters. Neither method is a good practice. How does one solve this dilemma?

One way is to adopt what might be termed the general "theory of acceleration" regarding study time. Essentially, this theory advocates starting slowly in the beginning (e.g., keeping up with reading assignments and homework) and increasing the amount and intensity of studying as the test draws nearer. This concept allows you to have some free time for other activities during the early "inter-test period" and avoids the panic reaction experienced by the perennial procrastinator. Although this schedule requires more discipline than other, less desirable study techniques, it will provide you with a better lifestyle in the long run and will, believe it or not, improve your overall performance on test day.

TEACHER INTERACTION

Although this may surprise you, one of the best untapped resources in many college courses is the professor. It is to your advantage to seek out the help of your professor whenever you have a question.

There are several reasons for adopting this strategy and becoming acquainted with your class instructor. First, your professor can be an invaluable help to understanding the basics of the course upon which everything else is built. Also, many professors enjoy interacting with students on a personal basis and may favor those who visit with them, either consciously or subconsciously, with little tidbits of information that could be useful at test time.

Before you know it you will need those important letters of recommendation for medical school, and they will be all the better if you have fostered a personal relationship with your professors. In some cases you may be fortunate enough to develop a close lifelong friendship with your professor.

OTHER ASSIGNMENTS

In addition to exams, there are often other major assignments in individual courses. The two most common are term papers and special research/presentation projects. The most important concept to remember regarding these is to make sure your professor approves of your ideas or topic. One of the saddest examples of failure to do this is a student who wrote a brilliant paper (even the professor admitted it was excellent) for a history class but did not receive a passing grade because his topic was not included in the list provided at the beginning of the semester.

If you discuss your idea for the paper or project with your professor, he or she may have some materials or ideas that you can use. In this way your professor will feel more involved in your project, and this may be an asset in the final evaluation of it (i.e., your grade). Finally, try to start your paper or project early, as a late start doesn't allow you to get your professor's help and hasty writing will probably be less than your best. It can also interfere with study time that could be better spent preparing for final exams.

CONTINGENCIES

A key concept to remember is *seek help early*. If the first quiz or test does not go well, it is imperative that you meet with your professor to discuss how to improve your performance. There is very little you or your professor can do the day before your final exam when 900 out of a possible 1,000 points have been completed and you have 420 points (i.e., you're going to fail no matter how you do on the final). Seeking assistance will help your performance and show your professors you care about their class. When final grades are due, if you happen to be on the borderline of a grade, they might be more apt to "bump you over."

An issue previously discussed was dropping a class. Before you decide to drop a class, be certain you know how this will appear on your final transcript. At some schools, if you drop a class by a certain date, such as at or around the time of the first test, the drop will not appear on your transcript. Remember, every school has different guidelines, so be sure to check the rules. The best scenario is to study and avoid dropping a class.

KNOW YOUR NUMBERS

Knowing where you stand in a class at any time during a semester is important for several reasons. Emotionally it keeps you "pumped up" for the long haul, because you know exactly what you need to do to get the grade you want. It also helps you set individual goals for the semester. For example, if you know you need a 95 percent on a term paper to keep you in contention for an "A," you will be more apt to start early and do your best work.

Knowing where you stand in each class will help you keep your priorities in order. For instance, if you were taking three classes and just prior to final exams you had a low "B" in one, a borderline "A"/"B" in another, and a strong "A" in the third, obviously your priorities would be to keep your strong "A," pull up your borderline grade, and preserve your "B." If you did not know these numbers before finals week, you would not be able to adopt a reasonable strategy for budgeting your time and energy to obtain these goals. So remember, know your numbers.

You must never forget that your primary objective in school is to learn. Never again (whether you make it into medical school or not) will you have the uninterrupted opportunity to study the variety of topics and areas available to you during your college years. Realize that doing well is important, but try not to sacrifice your learning opportunities by becoming overly grade-conscious.

Many people in medical school are illiterate in anything outside of medicine because they overloaded in the sciences while in college at the expense of their intellectual and personal growth in other areas. Following the guidelines in this chapter will help you get good grades and allow you the pleasure of learning. You won't regret it!

CHAPTER 9

PART-TIME JOBS

**"It is not enough to be busy . . . the question is:
what are we busy about?"**

Henry David Thoreau

You have a lot of studying to do! So much that you cringe at the idea of a part-time job. Do not. Having a job during college is important. It shows you are capable of getting excellent grades and working. It demonstrates your ability to budget time and work with people. These are skills that are needed for success in medical school and as a practicing physician.

A variety of positions exist. Many students find employment at their college, in government work-study positions, as cafeteria employees, or as security guards. Although any job is a good idea, certain occupations may enhance your chances of getting into medical school.

PARAMEDICAL POSITIONS

Selection committees often look for paramedical experience. Although such employment will not get you into medical school, it can give you an edge. Basically, there are eight opportunities available to you in medicine. These are positions as a phlebotomist, EKG technician, diener, EMT, orderly, nurse's aide, clerical worker, and volunteer. Each has advantages and disadvantages. There is also an appropriate time to consider each of these positions.

Early in your college career is not the time to look for a part-time job that requires regular hours. Employment as a phlebotomist, EKG technician, diener, EMT, orderly, nurse's aide, or clerical worker demands regular hours. You would be expected to be present every day you are assigned, despite the fact that you have an all-important inorganic chemistry exam the next day. These semiprofessional positions in the freshman year are to be avoided, since the risk of damaging your grade on exam day is not worth the experience you will garner.

In the freshman year, if you want hospital experience, a volunteer position would be appropriate. It should require only about one evening a week, preferably Friday or Saturday, so that at no time will it interfere with your study schedule. The best volunteer positions are usually found in the Emergency Department. Here you will learn to deal with families in crisis situations. Some hospitals will actually allow you to work with patients in the emergency room. This is excellent training. You will see how doctors, nurses, and technicians interact. You will also learn some medical vocabulary, which will make your third year of medical school easier. If an emergency position is not available, look for positions in critical care areas such as the Intensive Care Unit or Renal Dialysis Unit. However, any position will be better than no position at all, so take what you can get.

If you are not involved with repeating inorganic chemistry or auditing organic chemistry the summer after your freshman year, opportunities for employment exist. Now is the time to consider a summer job that will place you in either a hospital or nursing home environment. Look for jobs as an orderly, nurse's aide, or clerical worker. Place applications in early March or April, as these positions are often difficult to find. Your volunteer experience may help you get your foot in the door. Once again, put a high priority on positions in critical care areas. A job as an orderly or nurse's aide is probably best. A job as a clerical worker will teach medical vocabulary and enhance your ability to talk to people with problems.

Although they provide the best experience, some positions take too much training for a three-month job. In addition, employers usually expect a long-term job commitment. A position as a phlebotomist, EKG technician, diener, or EMT should probably be deferred until the end of your sophomore year. These positions will offer you full-time employment for the summer and extend into your junior and senior year, which can mean spending your summers in the same city as your college. Positions like these may prove to be an excellent addition to your medical school application, as the skills learned will be useful in medical school.

All of the positions mentioned are difficult to secure. You must complete a one- to twelve-week training course. Prior hospital experience will increase your chances of securing one of these positions, but you will also have to be aggressive and start your search in March or April of your sophomore or junior year.

Of the four positions just mentioned, perhaps the best for a college student is phlebotomist. Training takes one to two weeks. As a phlebotomist, you will learn to draw venous and arterial blood samples. This skill will be helpful in your junior and senior years of medical school as well as during your internship. The phlebotomist position is an opportunity to familiarize yourself with most of the blood tests, their normal values, and the time necessary to process the tests. You will spend a significant amount of time talking to patients, which is an important skill to acquire. Probably, you will have an opportunity to get to know a pathologist who might provide you with a letter of recommendation to medical school. This could really help!

Another good opportunity is a position as an EKG technician. These technicians run heart rhythm strips on patients. Training takes one to two weeks. You will again have the opportunity to spend a significant amount of time with patients. In addition, with a little extra work you can learn basic rhythm abnormalities, which is an essential skill for a medical student and physician. You will also have the opportunity to get to know a cardiologist, which presents an opportunity for a letter of recommendation. If you do get a job as an EKG technician, spend two afternoons reading *Rapid Interpretation of EKG's* by Dale Dubin, M.D. (Cove's Publishing). This is a quick way to learn to recognize most of the basic EKG abnormalities and will make your time spent as an EKG technician more challenging and educational.

A job as a diener is very much respected in the medical community. Training is on the job. These individuals act as autopsy assistants to pathologists. Since most hospitals do not do that many autopsies, this is a position that requires an on-call status. You will usually carry a pager and be contacted when an autopsy is to be done. As this position is usually part-time, you can often work in another position in the hospital while staying on call as a diener. Because the hours are difficult to manage (a call can come in at any time of day or night), this can be a demanding job, but it is interesting and educational. In the silent atmosphere of an autopsy room you will learn to confront the stark reality of death and disease.

One of the best positions is employment as an Emergency Medical Technician (EMT). These individuals staff ambulances. Getting a position in this area will take some extra work on your part. The summer after your freshman year or second semester sophomore year, look for an evening EMT training class. They meet one to two nights a week for two to three hours and last 8 to 12 weeks. Training classes are usually taught by trade schools or the local ambulance service. The easiest way to find out about these courses is to call your community's ambulance service. This activity requires planning on your part to avoid interference with class work. You should probably look into local training during your freshman year so that when time permits, you can take the class work. The course is usually inexpensive, not too difficult, and highly educational. Of all the possible health-related jobs you can get, an EMT position probably provides the best learning experience. It does, however, require the most work to secure. Even if you never work as an EMT, taking the classes and certification exam are worthwhile for the credentials. This will also enhance your chances of securing other hospital positions.

NONMEDICAL POSITIONS

Although working in a health care setting is desirable, the most important aspect of any experience is the opportunity to learn to interact with people. Not only is this important to your future success in the health care field, it is also something medical school admission committees consider.

There are many non–health care activities that fit this category. Some examples include restaurant hosts, tour guide attendants, sales representatives, and management positions in small shops. A unique, interesting, and well-paying job one author held was as a disc jockey/dance host for parties and weddings. The work involved playing taped music, running lights, and coordinating events such as weddings, company parties, and reunions. Not only did it require nerves of steel to deal with brides and company presidents, but also finesse and charisma to make sure everyone had a good time. This job taught valuable lessons in communication, time management, and patience. Several times during medical school interviews, dance host experiences were discussed. Interesting and sometimes humorous stories about various job experiences can improve your ability to express yourself in times of stress. That ability can be valuable in the interview setting.

Keep in mind that, although working in the health care field is desirable, any job that will develop your communication and/or coping skills is important. Employment that interests you, challenges you, and in the process makes you a better medical school candidate should be your ultimate goal.

Securing employment is very important to your career plans. Working will teach you to deal with patients and can give you contacts that will enhance your chances of getting into medical school. If your job is a health care position, it will also demonstrate to admissions committees that you know something about a medical career. Finding a position, however, takes careful planning. Always take a job in which you can excel. If you are busy with classes, getting good grades must come first. However, if it is a choice between more play time versus working, know where your priorities are and find that job! If you are considering a health care position, always apply at several hospitals and for different positions, because openings are difficult to find, especially if you are willing to work only weekends. Remember, holding a part-time job is important to your application to medical school.

CHAPTER 10

COLLEGE ACTIVITIES

"If I had my life to live over, I'd try to make more mistakes next time. I would relax. I would limber up. I would be sillier than I have been this trip. I know of few things I would take seriously. I would be crazier. I would be less hygienic. I would climb more mountains, swim more rivers, and watch more sunsets. I would eat more ice cream and less beans. I would have more actual troubles and fewer imaginary ones. You see, I am one of those people who live sensibly and sanely, hour after hour, day after day. Oh, I have had my moments, and, if I had it to do over again, I'd have more of them. In fact, I'd try to have nothing else. Just moments, one after another, instead of living so many years ahead each day. I have been one of those people who never go anywhere without a thermometer, a hot-water bottle, a gargle, a raincoat, and a parachute. If I had to do it over again, I would go places and do things and travel lighter than I have. If I had my life to live over, I would start barefooted earlier in the spring and stay that way later in the fall. I would play hooky more, I wouldn't make such good grades except by accident. I would ride on more merry-go-rounds. I'd pick more daisies."

Nadine Star

53

Your free time is severely limited. As a premed it is difficult to achieve a proper balance between work and play. You will be tempted to devote all your free time to textbooks. This will not, however, make you a good medical school applicant or physician. You must find ways to acquire people skills that are not found in textbooks. Like most college students, you will be tempted to spend your spare time partying or dating. Although this may be your preferred lifestyle, it will not win points with the medical school selection committee. If you are interested in going to medical school, your playtime must be strategically planned.

In three to four years, when you are filling out your medical school application form, two blank spaces will read "Honors Received While in College" and "Extracurricular, Community, and/or Avocational Activities While in College or After." Although there are only five blank lines, they will grow precipitously in magnitude if you do not fill them in. The solution: Get involved!

Almost any activity will do; however, some are better than others. Selection committees like to see activities that encourage good written and oral communication skills. Awards and honors that confirm your abilities are great additions to your credentials.

SPEECH TEAM

One good activity is membership on a speech team. Even if you did not actively participate in speech or debate in high school, speech coaches are usually obligated to give you a chance to attend tournaments. Writing one speech a year can easily be done during the summer. It can then be used for the entire competitive season. Coaches will usually allow you to select the tournaments you attend. Being away from campus two to three Saturdays a semester is usually not too much of a burden on any premed's schedule. As most tournaments have beginners' divisions, you may win awards, even if you are inexperienced. You will be surprised how much public speaking will help you in future interviews and presentations in classes, medical school, and medical practice.

You should consider participating in "informative" or "demonstration" speech events. These will be the most helpful in improving presentation skills. Another event, called "impromptu," gives you three minutes to prepare a three- to five-minute talk on a subject you are assigned. Often these topics are abstract questions such as "Why is snow white?" or they may ask you to address a question such as "What is the most important constitutional freedom: life, liberty, or the pursuit of happiness?" If this sounds difficult, it is. But it is an area of speech in which you can compete with little preparation and offers you excellent training in learning to respond to interview questions, which ultimately will help you get into medical school, no matter how much embarrassment you are forced to endure to get there. If speech is an interest, contact your college speech coach, who will be happy to discuss the various speech events and give you ideas for possible topics.

If competitive speech is unavailable at your college, consider joining Toastmasters. This is a private organization that holds weekly meetings for the sole purpose of practicing speaking skills. Many members have little or no speaking experience so no matter how poor your speaking skills, you will fit in.

INTERNATIONAL RELATIONS CLUB

If you are interested in international politics, your school's International Relations Club may be of interest. It provides an opportunity to learn how other countries think about various issues and provides you with an opportunity to give speeches as well as defend your position in front of a large group of people. Each IRC event involves several colleges throughout the United States, giving you the opportunity to travel and to meet students from other institutions. As the college usually provides funding to attend IRC tournaments, it is an inexpensive way to travel to new cities, meet new people, and develop skills that will be useful when you apply to medical school. If you are interested in the International Relations Club, membership information can usually be obtained through your college political science or history department.

PREMEDICAL CLUBS

Joining a premedical club is a good idea. Often these clubs will have a number of upperclassmen in them who can assist you in selecting future science courses. They may also have test files that can make your life a little bit easier. If your school does not have a premedical club, consider starting one. It is fairly easy to have one meeting a month. Meetings usually consist of inviting a local physician to speak for 15 minutes on "My Specialty." As there are well over 30 medical specialties, you can keep the program active for over a year. It is a good idea to invite your school's premedical advisor or the local dean of a medical school. Both of these individuals are people you really want to meet. To make it easier for them, prepare a list of questions you are interested in having addressed. They will be more apt to come if they do not have to take the time to prepare a lecture.

SCIENCE CLUBS

Other organizations of interest are biology, physics, and chemistry clubs. As you probably will want to take a few extra upper-division courses, membership in these clubs will give you a chance to talk to upperclassmen intimately familiar with most of the courses you are considering. Access to test files may be a rewarding plus to a one-hour meeting once a month.

POLITICAL OFFICES

Running for a school office is educational. However, you must be careful about position selection. Being president of the student body is a tremendous honor, but the amount of free time consumed may be disproportional to the enjoyment you receive from filling this position. A more appropriate political position to seek may be filling a representative position on the student council or your dorm floor. You should also look for positions that will put you in contact with prominent members of your college, such as the dean or college president. For example, being a member of the college fund-raising committee or alumni association may put you in contact with individuals who can help meet your future need for letters of recommendation. Medical school selection committees often consider political association as demonstration that you get along with your peers. It also demonstrates you have an outgoing personality, another attribute medical school selection committees consider. Political positions require that you give speeches; consequently you will have an opportunity to improve your oral communication skills.

TEAM SPORTS

Playing team sports demonstrates you are a "team player," which is a quality a medical student and doctor must have. However, you must select the sport discreetly. Joining a basketball team that practices four hours a day is not conducive to studying or preparing for exams. Always remember to weigh the benefit of the activity against the possible consequences to your grade point average.

RESEARCH PROJECTS

An interesting and rewarding activity is a research project with a professor. This may involve three to six credit hours and give you an opportunity to co-author a published paper. However, do not be taken in. Almost all professors are looking for free help. You must find one that publishes papers regularly so that you will reap the benefits of your labors. This is also a good way to get to know a science teacher. As you will be needing two science letters of recommendation, a wise choice may be an instructor you enjoy and in whose class you were academically successful. Medical selection committees are usually made up of research scientists, so having a research project while in college will be a valuable addition to your list of credentials.

CONTESTS

On most campuses, many departments and companies sponsor writing contests. Although time consuming, spending a Christmas vacation putting together a paper may be worth your time, especially if you are fortunate enough to win. This is another opportunity to fill the awards space that might otherwise be very blank.

There are many activities on most college campuses. The most important concept is finding an activity of interest and staying involved. Some activities are better than others. Look every one over, keeping in mind that you must constantly weigh the time necessary to participate against any possible detrimental effects it may have on your grade point average. You cannot afford to not be involved. Being a good doctor requires more than intelligence; you must acquire the social skills necessary to deal with people.

CHAPTER 11

APPLICATION FORMS

"Accurst ambition, How dearly I have bought you."

J. Dryden

If you have been strategically planning your career for the last three years, your medical school application is nothing to fear. You have prepared your credentials to meet the requirements of the American Medical College Application Service (AMCAS) form that now sits in front of you.

You have impressive awards and honorary society memberships to put in the "Honors Received While in College" section. You have been active in a variety of on- and off-campus activities, demonstrating your ability to work with and lead others, and can easily fill in the "Extracurricular, Community and/or Avocational Activities While in College or After" section. Since you have worked in various jobs, including at least one in a hospital, you have a list for the "Employment During Current School Year" and "Employment During Previous School Years" blanks. You have spent some of your summer vacation time volunteering, taking an EMT class, taking a trip to a foreign country, or working with a local physician, so you can comfortably answer the question "How have you spent your summers during your college years?"

If you have selected your classes carefully and given all your classes your best effort, you should have an outstanding grade point average to calculate. Since you studied for the MCAT the first time, you will be able to answer "one" to the question, "Number of MCATS taken."

59

The answers to all these questions have taken planning, hard work, and stamina. The reward for your efforts will be a positive demonstration to medical schools that you are both a good student and a well-rounded individual with a diversity of interests and talents and the necessary communication skills to become a good physician.

The final challenge of the AMCAS application is the "Personal Comments" section. There is room for an 800- to 900-word essay, giving you the opportunity to demonstrate to each medical school admissions committee why you should be selected. Most students combine an autobiography with an explanation of their desire to go to medical school. An effort should be made to incorporate some of your important accomplishments, interesting employment, activities that demonstrate communication and leadership skills, and unique qualities that make you a positive addition to a medical school class and the medical profession. You should also discuss the considerations and reasons you have for pursuing a medical career. How did you develop an interest in medicine? Is your decision to pursue medicine based on realistic criteria? How have you prepared yourself?

Summarizing your life in 800 to 900 words is a major challenge. It takes time and energy to develop a well-written, grammatically correct, neatly typed personal statement. When you finish your rough draft, you should have as many people as possible proofread it. When you are satisfied with the finished product, it is a good idea to find an English professor to give it a final review. The typing should be accurate. Complete a practice draft first to assure that it will fit between the margins of the AMCAS form. When you are ready for the final draft, either find a typist who can produce it error free or enter it accurately into a word processor and use a letter-quality printer that will allow perfect reproduction. With the modern typing/printing equipment available, an error-free draft is the standard. Nothing shatters an application more quickly than a spelling or grammar error picked up by one of your interviewers. You may consider spelling and grammar to be trivial; however, as a physician, a misplaced decimal point on a prescription can cause tragic results. Reviewers have a justifiable reason to question your attention to detail!

Treat your personal comments as the most important statement you have ever written. Start several months before the due date and concentrate on careful preparation. The final draft should be letter perfect!

On the following pages are five exact reproductions of actual medical students' "Personal Comments" sections sent in to the AMCAS. They are illustrations and should not be considered the ideal. Your personal

statement should reflect your own unique qualities and not be a copy of
the work of others. Information identifying the authors of the following
"Personal Comments" sections has been changed. A critique following
each "Personal Comments" section will help identify errors.

Personal Comments, Student A

There is more to a doctor than intelligence. In modern American it is important that he or she also have the personability
to converse with and understand people from diverse cultures.
He must have an intense zeal to explore new material yet the
common cense to direct some energy to arts, sports, and
hobbies. Overall, I think he must be dedicated to the betterment of the world through direct action with people; it should
be a vocation, not a job. I hope that my action, interests and
philosophy prove that medicine is the natural next step in my
life.

I lived on the west coast of America for the first seven
years of my life and the next eleven in Holten, a tiny fishing
village of five hundred people on the northern coast of Ire-
land. I completed my six years in the village National School,
two years of secondary level in a Carmal boarding school, and
the last three in a nearby Christian Youths' School. During my
Irish years, I ran cross-country for the school and town and
helped form an athletic club in our village, becoming its first
chairman and trainer. Each summer I took the Irish Water
Safety Association's Life Saving courses and taught the children to swim. I found great satisfaction in the less informal
activities of canoeing, hiking and sailing.

In the summer of 1979, my parents bought a house in
Hingham, Massachusetts, and I moved over to start college.
The other six members of our family joined me the following
summer. In the interim, I invited a family of homeless Viet-
namese boat people to share our new (300 year old) house
with me. Since then, I have completed the U.S. Marine Corps
Platoon Leaders' Class Program, graduating as honor man in
my platoon. I taught Contraternity of Christian Doctrine to first
graders for a year, and Christian Youth Organization (CYO)
since then, acting as academic and spiritual coordinator. I am
interested in the theater and in classical as well as modern

music and literature. I have participated in the Outing Club's canoeing, climbing and winter camp trips and am helping to get authorization for a campus scuba club.

As a freshman marine biology major and journalism minor, I worked on the Northern News' staff for the first semester and became Arts and Entertainment Editor the second. In my sophomore year I was elected vice-president of the Chemistry Club, becoming president in my junior year and being invited into the honorary fraternity, Tau Pi Sigma. I've been tutoring general chemistry for the past three semesters and working for the Chemistry Department for two. In my senior year I am working for the Chemistry Department, tutoring, teaching CYO, working as an emergency room volunteer at Mass General, and doing research in the Department of Neurology, Harvard School of Medicine, in the area of cyclic AMP, specifically, the guanyl nucleotide-binding unit (G-unit) of the system.

I came to a major in marine biology because it seems to provide a natural combination of my interests in the outdoors, the sea, and with scientific inquiry. In my sophomore year however, I began to reflect on my courses in terms of my interests in their content and their connection to a life's vocation. I changed to biochemistry for I discovered that it lay closer to my real interest. It is more precise, it answers more questions and delves more deeply into the knowledge of human science; it is challenging.

But as yet, I had not connected my divergent interests to an occupation that would give adequate expression to my commitment to scientific training and my desire to be of service to others. I wanted a vocation that would concentrate my energies into a field where my intellectual, spiritual and physical needs could find fulfillment.

When my advisor, Dr. Pittner, first mentioned medicine to me in the latter part of my sophomore year, I recognised immediately that the profession of medicine is a logical choice for someone with my background and interests. The more I read and talked to people about the life of a physician, the more the study of medicine excites me. I am not deterred by prospects of a gruelling physical routine or the lack of leisure time. I recognize that arduous study, long hours, physical exertion, emotional and mental strain and moral and legal

responsibility are part of the medical student's, and later the
doctor's daily existence. I am excited by the opportunity to
deal with people, to solve problems and to continue the learning process.

I see medicine as a humane branch of science in which my
need for continued study will find its fulfillment in the con-
crete problems of my patients and its motive for and test of
success of my ability to help solve their problems. Such a life
appeals to me very strongly.

CRITIQUE

This "Personal Comments" section is very interesting. The author has
been involved in many impressive activities and incorporates many of
the concepts previously discussed, combining a short autobiography, personal philosophy, and reasons for his suitability for medical school.

However, this statement demonstrates a number of errors you should
avoid. There are numerous errors in spelling, grammar, syntax, and punctuation, all of which should be corrected. In the first paragraph, for example, the author switches pronouns abruptly from "he or she" to "he"
without explanation. Awkward word choices also detract from the
applicant's statement. "Flexibility" is clearer and works better than
"personability"; instead of " . . . the betterment of . . . ," the word "improving" is concise and active. Likewise, "prove that medicine is . . . "
would be clearer and more emphatic as "prove medicine to be . . . ."
"American," "cense," and "action" are all incorrect; they should be
"America," "sense," and "actions," respectively. Finally, in order to maintain stylistic consistency with the rest of the text, a comma should follow
"interests."

The second paragraph leaves us wondering just how many times the
applicant needed to take the Irish Water Safety Association's Life Saving
course. He probably found canoeing, hiking, and sailing to be "less formal" instead of "less informal."

The humor in the third paragraph is good: "our new (300 year old)
house." However, the expression "moved over" is clearer as "I moved
back to the United States." The author should explain the significance of
the various positions, awards, and organizations he mentions (e.g., platoon honor man). He should also watch for stylistic inconsistencies that
disrupt the flow of his statement ("I am interested in the theater . . . "
among a litany of accomplishments).

In the fourth paragraph, the contraction "I've" is too informal for a "Personal Comments" section. The author switches tense in the middle of the paragraph without a proper segueway. In addition, we are never told what college the author actually attends.

At the beginning of the fifth paragraph, "I chose a major" would be more specific than "I came to . . . ." " . . . it seems," then would become "it seemed" for correct verb tense. There should be commas inserted after "In my sophomore year" and "it answers more questions . . ."; a colon or em dash should offset the final clause ("it is challenging"), not a semi-colon. The causitive "for" is too formal for this essay; it should be "because." "But" should be eliminated at the beginning of the sixth paragraph.

In the seventh paragraph "Dr. Pittner" should have a first name. Sequence of tenses should be followed; "excited" is required after "read and talked."

The concluding paragraph is not coherent. There should be a period after "patients." The next sentence could read, "The profession will test my ability to solve my patients' problems, one of my motives for choosing medicine."

Personal Comments, Student B

A medical doctor requires a person who has a diverse background; adapts to new situations quickly, enjoys learning, reading and hard work; and accepts responsibility. In addition, he or she must be: inquisitive, able to ask the right question at the right time; perceptive, listening and learning from each new situation; and most important, persuasive, enjoying informing others and helping them to understand, accept, and follow his instructions. It is my belief that I will bring to the medical profession these requirements.

I was raised on a farm near Blue Hill, Nebraska, an agricultural community. My father is a farmer and has been actively engaged in the development, production, and processing of hybrid milo and corn. My mother, formerly a teacher, is now a homemaker. I have one younger brother.

Attending a small rural high school, I had the opportunity to pursue many interests. I participated in football, basketball, debate, speech, drama, annual staff, choir, and band. Outside of school, I was actively involved in 4-H. One of my 4-H projects, raising purebred cattle, allowed me to finance much of my college education. I also enjoyed Demolay, an international young men's Christian organization and am a Past Master Counsilor of the Red Cloud Chapter.

As a student at the University of Nebraska—Lincoln I will be awarded a major in speech communications with supporting studies in science, business, and honors. Debate and speech teaches you to: think on your feet, organize your thoughts, react rapidly, and communicate effectively and precisely. As a debator for four years, I have addressed such topics as penal reform, national health insurance, unemployment and energy. This semester I have written a humorous after dinner speech. The skills I have learned will be especially important for a doctor, as one argument often wins a debate round, so too, choosing the right words may open the road to recovery. My science studies will help me grasp the technical aspects of medicine. Of special interest to me as an undergraduate was a course in human genetics. I especially enjoy genetics because it incorporates the problem-solving skills of physics and chemistry, and perhaps the very essence of biology as it attempts to decipher the "key to life." Last summer, because of my interest in this field, I did volunteer work in the Department of Genetics at UMMC. Medicine is a science, yet, it is also an art since ability to work with people, comprehend their problems, and understand their lives are an integral part of the healing process. As a doctor, I will have an understanding of many of my patients' problems because of the rational perspective on life my business course work has provided. Perhaps the most helpful program of study in this respect was being a member of the Nebraska Honors Program. This group of discussion classes represented an outstanding insight into political and social science, philosophy, literature, and theology.

Practical experience in a working environment is also important to development of a physician. Over the years I have financed my education and at the same time gained experience through working as a salesman, supervisor, law firm clerk, farmer, and phlebotomist. Farm work has helped to prepare me for a doctor's life, just as patient's do not always call between 9 and 5, farm animals tend to deliver when it is cold, wet, and muddy.

At the end of my junior year, I took a year off to finance the reminder of my education and make sure I was not suffering from the "Marcus Welby" syndrome in my desire to study medicine. Working as a phlebotomist helped me realize that medicine offers everything I desire in a profession. I especially enjoyed working in pediatrics, as I like children and the opportunity their care affords in the practice of preventive medicine.

As an individual I am usually good natured, except before chemistry exams, enjoy socializing with friends, and date often. My friends and professors describe me as zealous in arguments, inquisitive, and witty. My favorite activity is reading. In making my decision to study medicine, I have attempted to experience the profession vicariously in both its positive and negative aspects. Consequently, I have included in my medical reading such books as *The Clay Pedestal* and *The Education of a Medical Heretic*. I was impressed that the authors, even in their criticism of medical care, still held the ideals of the profession attainable. The medical profession will provide me with a constant exposure to new and interesting people, ideas, and challenges. It will allow me to do clinical research, teach, live in rural Nebraska, and still keep abreast with scientific thought. I believe I will make a good physician and practitioner of the art and science of medicine.

CRITIQUE

This student's "Personal Comments" follow a logical order. He includes an autobiography in which he attempts to incorporate his rationale for why the admissions committee should select him as a medical student and eventual physician. He believes the focus of his education and activities support the qualities he deems appropriate in a doctor.

There are a number of obvious errors in this personal statement. For one, the author could have benefitted from using a spell-check. In the first paragraph, the correct spelling is *perceptive*. In the third paragraph, the word is *counselor;* in the fourth, *debater;* in the fifth, *remainder*.

Likewise, the author does not seem to know exactly to whom he is referring. He should begin with, "The medical profession requires . . . ." In the second sentence he uses the pronouns "he or she," which inexplicably become "his" by the end of the sentence. Throughout the essay, the author also neglects to follow sequence of tenses—"I especially enjoy . . . " in the fourth paragraph, for example, should be "I especially *enjoyed*."

When preparing your personal statement, you should take time to carefully review punctuation, grammar, and word choices. The first sentence of the fourth paragraph should read " . . . I will be awarded a degree in speech communications with supporting studies . . . " The sentence beginning "The skills I have learned . . . " is a run-on sentence. There should be a period after "doctor." The next sentence should read: "As one argument often wins a debate round, so too, choosing the right words may open the road to recovery." Also, the paragraph is too long; it could be broken at "My science studies will help me . . . ." The organization, University of Minnesota Medical Center, should be written out.

In the fifth paragraph, the sentence "Farm work has helped me . . . " could be rewritten, "Farm work, in particular, has helped me to prepare for a doctor's life. Just as patients do not always call . . . ." In addition, "9 to 5" should be written out "nine to five."

Personal Statement, Student C

My purpose is to become a competent physician who is committed not only to the diagnosis and treatment of physical and mental disease, but to the improvement of medical care in our swiftly changing society. I think I am an intelligent, adaptive individual who has the motivation to manage the challenge of medicine.

Although my planned course to become a physician may be irregular, it has been advantageous. I pursued engineering because I wanted to learn a basic foundation of scientific knowledge and problem solving skills. To assure this, I supplemented my civil engineering and bioengineering curriculums with courses in biology, chemistry, accounting, and political science. I studied French to improve my communication skills. I became involved in student organizations—Epsilon Phi (pres., sec.), Society of Women Engineers (v. pres., sec., treas.), All University Fund (treas.), Kappa Delta Sorority (sec., pub. chair.)—to improve my leadership skills. I am currently completing a master's degree in bioengineering to strengthen my background in the biological sciences and to introduce me to subjects such as biomedical instrumentation and biomedical materials. Thus, my engineering education has established the basis for a solid career in medicine.

My decision to become a physician is well thought out and based on numerous discussions and experiences. I have talked with individuals working in many different areas of medicine, including rural health care and medical research. Many experiences have expanded my understanding of medicine:

Hospital Volunteer at The University of Virginia Hospital. I have observed patient care in many areas, such as plastic surgery, arthritis, and gynecology. Through close acquaintance with patients, I learned to appreciate their concerns and the value of effective physician–patient interaction.

Volunteer with Handicapped Individuals. Through the YMCA I taught retarded children to swim. I experienced the rewards and frustrations of teaching physically impaired individuals a skill.

Research Assistant for the Department of Industrial and Operations Engineering. We are investigating the relationship between cumulative trauma disorders and repetitiveness, force, and postural attributes of industrial tasks. Through this experience, I have learned that many factors—some subtle—must be considered to alleviate a health problem.

Participant at Conference on Ethics, Humanism, and Medicine. My participation at several conferences has exposed me to many issues, including passive euthanasia, living wills, and fetal rights. The conference impressed upon me the importance of a physician's awareness of changes in societal values.

I think I possess many qualities necessary for a capable physician. I am a good listener who is sincerely concerned with people's needs. As demonstrated by my many leadership positions, I have the confidence to make decisions. Although I am a realist, I am creative and imaginative which gives me the ability to empathize with people.

My work needs to be challenging. I am well organized and self-disciplined. Although I work effectively independently, I know the importance of group participation. Especially through my work in an engineering design firm, I developed the skills to communicate and work in group situations.

Even though I am intensely involved in my work and studies, I realize the necessity of relaxation. During my free time I enjoy skiing, backpacking, playing the piano, and reading.

In conclusion, I think I have the physical and intellectual abilities to be a competent physician who is prepared to meet tomorrow's challenges. I not only think I have the capabilities, I intuitively feel that I will be a success.

CRITIQUE

This is a very well-written personal statement. The author obviously has a diverse and interesting background. She is not a typical applicant and does an excellent job communicating her varied background to its greatest advantage. She has groomed herself in many respects for the qualities a selection committee deems valuable: a caring personality as demonstrated by her volunteer activities, varied exposure to medical fields, and the ability to work with others. She also emphasizes her communications skills, a key consideration for any selection committee.

In the second paragraph, the applicant should spell out the titles she has had: vice-president, secretary, etc. In the following paragraphs where she lists her volunteer positions, she should underline the positions: <u>Volunteer with Handicapped Individuals</u>.

There are a few problems with her presentation. She could have been more firm in her convictions, striking phrases such as "I think I" and simply stating "I am." Much to the author's credit, there are no spelling errors.

Personal Statement, Student D

My intention in pursuing a medical career is to be persistent. I have applied to medical school in the past and will continue to upgrade my credentials, maintain my commitment, and reapply with the hopes that one school will offer me an acceptance. I greatly encourage you to grant me an interview in order to find out my qualities, abilities, and aspirations in becoming a physician.

When reviewing my AMCAS application, one cannot help notice a deficiency in my scholastic records. If it wasn't for minority programs, I feel my chances in becoming a physician would be hopeless. Being of a minority is a struggle to better your life as well as the lives of your people. I would like to work for my people as a physician and show them it is possible for social mobility in professional careers. I applaud your Affirmative Action's program in its ability to let us improve our lives.

My qualifications are commented in the following paragraphs:

During my first year of college, I was enrolled in a Physics class, composed almost entirely of Juniors, and a General Chemistry class. I was unaccustomed to living in that particular environment and high level of competitive studying. Possessing a poor science background and a lack of proper guidance and counseling, I went through a dramatic year of receiving grades, which up to that point of my life, were disastrous. I sank into an attitude that I couldn't do better than "C" work and spent my first two years in college not believing that I could do well in school.

In my third year, still with the underlying desire to be a physician, I worked as an ACTION volunteer at a local Community Clinic, a low cost clinic for the indignant. During this time, I was exposed to physicians and other medical professionals which made a strong impact on me. I was able to have physicians and student physicians as influential friends and acquaintances. I felt purposefull in my position at the clinic and became determined to be a physician. I worked hard in the second half of my undergraduate years. During my last year, I worked as a Biochemistry research assistant at UCLA. The research, under the direction of Dr. William Scott, dealt with the role of pyruvate kinase in carcinoma cells. My grades have shown improvement where I was able to maintain a "B" science average during my last two years. I graduated with Bachelor Degrees in Sociology and Biological Sciences.

I was interested in Sociology because it is a science dealing with social behavior. I believe that a physician should understand the social, as well as the physical facets of an individual when treating him. Medicine is a trusting relationship between physicians and their patients. In dealing with patients of various racial and social cultures, it is imperative to know how to present one's self in order to initiate and uphold a professional relationship.

From the standpoint of my nonacademic medical qualifications, I believe I am an excellent applicant. I have had a number of leadership and philanthropist roles ranging from the Health Services Coordinator at the Community Clinic to being a teachers aid at a preschool. I have worked with many age groups and can take charge of a situation and make decisions.

My plans for this academic year is to study in UNDA Post-Baccalaureate premedical program for disadvantaged students. Every year they accept up to twenty students of which they feel are potential medical students. They have been able to boast a 75–80% medical acceptance level from their program. I am honored to be selected in this program and will work hard in order to become a physician.

CRITIQUE

This student makes a valiant attempt to turn her poor academic background to her advantage. Throughout the personal statement she reiterates her determination to continue to apply to medical school until she succeeds. Despite her strong ambition, it is apparent that her statement could have been significantly improved.

In the first paragraph the use of "persistent" is unclear; the writer appears to want to emphasize her intention to persist in her efforts until she attains a medical degree. "Encourage" in the second sentence should be "urge." The second paragraph is ambiguous in its intent. It needs to be rewritten to make its purpose clear: "Being a member of a minority engages you in a struggle to better your own life and can motivate you to want to improve the lives of your people as well. I would like to work for my people as a physician and show them it is possible for them to have social mobility through professional careers." Choosing the subject of a sentence and making complete statements is important.

In the fourth paragraph, "Physics" and "General Chemistry" should not have been capitalized. In the third sentence the tone is uneven. It would be preferable to say " . . . I went through a year in which my grades were the worst of any I'd ever received in my life. I became depressed by the idea that I could do no better than 'C' work, an attitude that stayed with me throughout my first two years in college."

Throughout the text, word misuse is a problem. For example, in the fifth paragraph, the author must have meant "indigent" rather than "indignant." The paragraph also illustrates the importance of checking the spelling of all words. At the end of the paragraph the sentence should read, "I graduated with Bachelor's degrees in Sociology and Biological Sciences." In the sixth paragraph, "one's self" should be "oneself." In the seventh paragraph the author illustrates the need to use the correct word form, as "philanthropist" should have been "philanthropic"; in the same sentence the position is "teacher's aide."

In the final paragraph, the author needs to use the correct subject form. For example, "My plans . . . is . . . " should be "My plan . . . is . . . ," as she has only one program. "Of which" should be "whom." "Able to boast" would be better as "can claim . . . ."

This personal statement illustrates the importance of proper use of words, spelling, grammar, and punctuation. Remedial assistance from a teacher or counselor could have helped eliminate the need for repeated applications.

Personal Statement, Student E

As a high school senior and concurrent student at UC, I developed an interest in medicine from my leisure readings in scientific literature. Besides being one of the most rapidly expanding fields on the scientific frontier, medicine attracted me because of its dedication to the well-being of all peoples, its discoveries intended only for constructive use.

During the past two years, I participated in two research projects, the first as a laboratory helper running a computer and assisting human subjects in a nutritional research investigation. As an engineering honor student, I was able to secure a position in the Department of Mechanical Engineering helping to carry out an experiment to study the transient response to mammalian heart tissues to varying levels of glycerol, an experiment in cryobiology that will later be published. Being exposed to research has been a valuable learning experience because unlike solving typical problem sets that call for only one method, I found that I had to think with an open mind. Whether it was designing a leakproof assemblage of tubes with limited material or determining the concentration of glycerol in a saline solution, I was able to tackle each problem by considering as many angles of approach as possible in order to avoid becoming entrapped in one mode of thought. Besides having the opportunity to try my own ideas, it was exciting to see the concepts that I had learned in theory, apply in practice. It also gives me pride and satisfaction to think that I may have been contributing to an increased understanding of human nutrition or towards a better way of preserving human organs for transplantation.

As well as disciplining myself mentally, I learned to discipline myself physically and took up handball in my freshman year. With constant practice, I became skilled in the game and, during this past year, earned fourth place in the Western Divisional Intercollegiate Championship and second in consolation at the national Intercollegiate Tournament in Memphis. Being in athletic competition has taught me the importance of being persistant and patient in achieving any goal.

To become acquainted with the medical field, I volunteered in an emergency ward at a local hospital during the past three years. As a volunteer, the most rewarding experiences came as a result of being in direct contact with patients. At times, I would leave the hospital numbed by experiences such as seeing a young boy weakened and emaciated by cancer, or watching a woman break down into tears when she learned that she may never walk again. It seemed so unfair that these individuals should have had to suffer when they did not choose nor deserve to have such misfortunes brought upon them. It is from these kinds of experiences that I have come to sense my own vulnerability and realize that it isn't only the patient's problem, it's also mine because of the fact that I'm human and not immune from debilitating accidents or diseases. Consequently, I have learned to develop sensitivities towards patients and their problems and have acquired some knowledge about the causes and treatments of their illnesses. It was gratifying to be able to provide these individuals with emotional support like giving reassurance to an aged woman who was about to undergo abdominal surgery for the second time, or clasping an infant's hands while the physician sutured a laceration. But I feel I have much more to offer in terms of scientific knowledge and diversity in contributing to the collective effort to bring these human problems under control, both in preventing their occurrence and in giving those, who have become victims, the opportunity to achieve the health that I have come to take for granted.

From my volunteer experiences, I have gained a sense of what it means to give unselfishly and derived much satisfaction from knowing that my efforts were put to good use. As a physician, it would give me the greatest satisfaction to know that my work is benefitting society, that future generations will be able to profit from it by enjoying the privilege of good health and that, someday, they may live the full potentials of their lifespans without having to confront crippling diseases and tragic mishaps that plague our world today. At present, I have not made up my mind as to whether I would pursue a research or a clinical career and, therefore, will leave my options open until something sparks my interest. Whether in research or in treating people directly, I feel that my background has made me mentally, physically, and emotionally prepared to commit my life to medicine and that I am eminently qualified for whichever pursuit I decide to undertake.

CRITIQUE

This is a well-written, well-organized, and interesting personal statement. The author makes a convincing argument as to why he should be selected. It is obvious that much time and energy went into the final draft as there is only one spelling error, "persistant," and few grammatical errors. He presents his employment history well, making it very clear that he has developed the "people skills" necessary to be a physician. It is also obvious that his understanding of the medical profession and his future role in it are well thought out. One cannot help feeling this individual will be a compassionate, caring physician.

Some of the following corrections should be made. In the first paragraph the name of the university should be written out. The last sentence would be improved by changing the end to " . . . all peoples, and its focus on discoveries intended only for constructive use." The second sentence in the second paragraph should read " . . . *of* mammalian heart tissue . . . ," and the next-to-last sentence should have " . . . applied in practice." The fourth paragraph is too long. The author might begin a new paragraph after " . . . misfortunes brought upon them."

Although it is easy to be critical of these personal comments, it is noteworthy that all the individuals that contributed these essays were accepted to several medical schools. As you complete your application, keep in mind how easy it was for these applicants to make errors in their personal statements. Some of the statements were read by several individuals and reviewed by English professors. The fact that errors escaped detection should encourage you to be very careful in completing your application.

The qualities and skills that these applicants emphasize include leadership, communication, responsibility, and compassion. All the applicants emphasize their understanding of the role of a physician and their own personal qualities that they perceive identify with this role.

The Personal Comments section of an application is an opportunity to err; therefore it is important that you prepare it carefully. Check, check, and check again. Start early and find several reviewers!

CHAPTER 12

THE MEDICAL COLLEGE ADMISSION TEST

"There are three categories of falsehood: lies, damn lies, and statistics."

Mark Twain

The most amazing statement ever heard from a medical school applicant is "I didn't study for the MCAT." Deans of medical schools are shocked by the rejected applicants who ask, "What can I do to improve my chances of getting in next year?" If MCAT scores were the obstacle, they indicate this and ask how much time the student spent preparing for the exam. The surprising response much of the time is "none." This strategy regarding the Medical College Admission Test is foolhardy.

The MCAT is one of the most important exams you will ever take. Most medical schools have a minimum cutoff score for acceptance and partially rank applicants based on these scores. It is the only way they have to compare you and the college you represent objectively against applicants from other institutions. Only a foolish premed would take an organic chemistry exam cold, so why do students think the MCAT can be faced without preparation?

FORMAT OF THE MCAT

The MCAT includes four basic tests: Physical Sciences, Biological Sciences, Verbal Reasoning, and a Writing Sample (essay). The test is an attempt to evaluate knowledge of basic concepts in biology, chemistry, and physics and to address problem-solving, critical thinking, and writing skills. The Verbal Reasoning section includes 65 multiple-choice questions based on 500 to 600 word reading passages. The Biological and Physical Sciences sections each consist of 77 multiple-choice questions. Each section includes 10 or 11 problem sets with 4 to 8 questions based upon the situations described. In addition each section includes approximately 15 questions that are independent of any passage. The Writing Sample consists of two 30-minute essays.

MCAT PREPARATION

Some students who do not prepare for the MCAT state they thought it was impossible to review four one-year science courses. This is ludicrous! In medical school you will probably be expected to take comprehensive exams covering the entire year at the end of each year and national boards covering all the material at the end of your sophomore and senior years. Very few medical students take and pass these exams without preparation. Most devote 4 to 12 weeks preparing for them. Not only is reviewing four courses manageable, it is a must!

Another argument, often heard from science majors, is that they have had numerous courses in these areas and do not think they need to review. Wrong again! The MCAT covers introductory-level course work in biology, inorganic chemistry, organic chemistry, and physics. The questions addressed on the MCAT can be answered based on this level of knowledge. Upper-division course work helps little, as inorganic chemistry concepts, for example, are covered only to a limited extent in upper-division chemistry classes and there are still many gaps in the presentation of inorganic chemistry principles. If you major in physics, you probably have not taken any more biology or chemistry courses than your nonscience-major counterparts. Finally, the MCAT is usually taken at the end of your junior year or early in your senior year, and it will have been two full years since you took most of this introductory-level course work. Not reviewing for this exam is taking an unnecessary risk!

One last argument is "If I don't do well, I will simply take it again." Unfortunately, medical schools receive copies of both of your MCAT scores. Some schools average the two scores; others take the lower of the two. Even if they use the higher score, both scores will be present in bold print on your AMCAS application. It is difficult to imagine a committee failing to notice that you did way below average the first time you took the test and only average the second time. Obviously, it is better to put your best foot forward the first time.

Whatever your excuse for not preparing for the MCAT, think again. If you really want to go to medical school, why take a chance? This exam should be considered equally important as the time and money you have devoted to your college career. If you are a borderline applicant, MCAT scores may make the difference between acceptance and rejection. If you are an outstanding student, MCAT scores may determine which medical schools accept you and what scholarships are provided.

WHEN TO TAKE THE MCAT

Deciding when to take the MCAT is difficult. Many students take the exam in the spring of their junior year. This allows one more opportunity to take the exam in the fall of your senior year should you not perform up to your expectations. It also allows you to apply for an early match position at your top choice and prevents you from missing the deadlines of a number of schools that require applications to be completed in the early fall. The major disadvantage is that it is difficult to prepare for this exam while classes are going on. If this is your choice, be prepared to cut your course load to 9 or 12 hours. You can always make up the time in a three-week presession or five-week summer session. Since you may be staying at school looking for a paramedical job, this can be an acceptable alternative.

Another option is to plan on spending the summer after your junior year preparing for the MCAT and working in a part-time or full-time job (medically oriented if possible). It will not be a fun summer, but neither is failing to meet your lifelong goal after working very hard to do well in all those previous classes.

MCAT REVIEW

There are basically two ways to prepare for the MCAT. If you are dedicated and extremely organized, you can review your textbooks and class notes. If you select this route, you must also review *several* practice test books. There are a number of excellent review books available. These books provide several examples of MCAT tests and discuss formats as well as strategies for improving your test scores. If you select this method of preparing for the exam, you must start early, as each sample test takes several hours. After you complete these exams, you will find your areas of weakness and need to concentrate your review efforts appropriately. Although college courses covered the fundamentals of biology, inorganic and organic chemistry, and physics, they did not teach you to work the types of problems the MCAT stresses. The MCAT places a premium on the rapid completion of problems. If you are unfamiliar with the instructions or question types, you may severely penalize yourself by not completing the test.

One challenge of the MCAT is the Verbal Reasoning section. Even if you have had many humanities courses, do not be overconfident. This section stresses questions that you may not have experienced. It is difficult to complete this section in the allotted time. Most students think this section is the easiest one on the MCAT. Actually, and much to their surprise, it is often the section with their lowest MCAT score. Most students miss only a few problems in this section but because it is scaled (everything is based on student performance), missing just a few questions may drastically lower your score.

The other option for MCAT preparation is to take a review course. There are several types available. The authors recommend the Stanley Kaplan Review; however, other excellent courses may be available in your area. Some colleges offer review courses. Mail-order versions are available. Tuition for review courses can be high, but is often little more than the cost of a single class in a private college or a little less than a semester at a public school. It may be a worthwhile investment for you. Courses often use tapes and lectures, covering every aspect of the MCAT. They give you a comprehensive review of pertinent course work and include numerous exams.

Studying for the MCAT is a test—a test of your willingness to put in the time necessary to assure your admission to medical school. It is also a test of your willingness to work and study on your own, independent of an instructor and a grade hanging over your head. As a physician you will be studying on your own for the rest of your life. Now is the time to establish your willingness to take the steps necessary to assure that MCAT scores are a help and not a hindrance in seeking acceptance into medical school.

CHAPTER 13

LETTERS OF RECOMMENDATION

"They never take the time to think about what
really goes on in those one-to-one sessions. They see
it as rape instead of seduction; they miss the elabo-
rate preparation that goes on before the act is
finally done."

Lyndon B. Johnson

One of the most important questions you will ever ask is "Will you please
write a letter of recommendation for me for medical school?" Obtaining
good letters of recommendation can be difficult, especially at a large
college that affords little opportunity to get to know your instructors on a
personal level. Getting a letter of recommendation requires a considerable amount of planning on your part.

Most medical schools require at least three letters of recommendation,
but you should arrange for five since some of them may be lost or not
written on time. Sending a few extra good recommendations can only
help. You may be required to obtain one to two from science instructors,
one to two from nonscience instructors, and one from a physician or
employer.

Some students obtain letters from politicians or individuals they believe to have influence, such as a state senator. With few exceptions, these
letters are a double-edged sword rather than a positive contribution to

your application. Politicians tend to be controversial individuals who are either well liked or much disliked. Selection committees may be composed of 10 or 12 individuals of diverse political outlooks. In other words, keep in mind JFK's quote "A man without enemies has no character" before asking your family's political friend for a letter of recommendation. The individual you select should be someone who knows you and is familiar with your personality, not someone repaying a favor for one of your family members.

Obtaining science letters can be difficult, especially for the nonscience major. Often basic science classes contain hundreds of students. If you are a nonscience major, you may find it hard to obtain a letter of recommendation from an instructor from whom you took only a one-semester class. After two years, the instructor will probably remember little about you, and your letter will be no more than a reiteration of the fact that you received a "B" on the first exam and improved considerably after that. There are several ways around this problem.

Make every effort to get to know your instructors. Sit in or near the front row and try not to miss class. If you have a question, ask it after class, when your instructor can recognize your face rather than a raised hand in a sea of noses. Every time you ask a question, first introduce yourself until you are remembered by name. Do not be afraid to discuss exam questions. Do not argue for points, but seek to understand the underlying concept. Do not criticize the test questions. Keep in mind who wrote them!

There is a fine line between knowing your professor and becoming a "brown noser." Do not cross it! Having worked with students for years, professors know the difference between an interested student and one who plays up to teachers. Do not become the latter. Always address instructors by their proper title. Do not use first names unless invited.

If one of your instructors is particularly good, and you did well in that instructor's introductory class, try to fit into your schedule one of his or her upper-division courses in your sophomore or junior year. Needless to say, work hard! You must impress this individual with your abilities if you want to get a sparkling letter of recommendation!

If you find instructors you enjoy talking to and who seem easy to work with, consider asking them if you can do a one- to three-credit-hour research project or directed readings with them in your sophomore or junior year. You may not have time for a lab project, but the instructor may be willing to set up a literature review on a specific topic. This will give you an opportunity to learn to read journal articles critically, and it is also a good way to get to know your instructor.

In addition to science letters of recommendation, you will need one or two letters from nonscience instructors. The same rules apply. If you find an instructor you really like, take several of his or her courses. You will probably learn the most from someone you like personally and will probably do your best in that instructor's classes.

A final letter of recommendation might come from one of your employers. If you can get to know a physician well, he or she would be a good choice. A letter indicating you are a hard worker and can work well with patients or people is important.

Before you ask for a letter of recommendation, you must be prepared. You should be ready to hand the individual you select a curriculum vitae, a copy of your personal statement, and, if your grades or MCAT results are excellent, a copy of your grades or scores. This will demonstrate your many strong points in addition to the fact that you did well in the instructor's class. Instructors may even include some of these points in their letters. They also separate you from all the other applicants for whom an instructor may be writing a letter of recommendation. The fact that you are unique, organized, and prepared may make the difference between a good letter of recommendation and an excellent one. Be positive and confident about being accepted, as your attitude may be reflected in the tone of a letter of recommendation.

Your request for a letter of recommendation should be made in September or early October of your senior year at the latest. Science instructors will soon be inundated with requests for letters. If this occurs, you might not end up getting as good a letter as you would have earlier in the year. As most medical schools process thousands of applications, you may find that one or more of your letters of recommendation might be lost by either the schools or the U.S. Postal Service. Schools will often delay examination of an applicant's file until it is complete, so make sure to call each school and confirm that all of your letters of recommendation have reached their destination.

Some colleges have medical school committees that prepare a letter of recommendation. If this is the case, make an effort to find out who the committee members are. If possible, take classes from them. At some schools, the committee determines who will be allowed to apply to medical school. If they refuse to write you a letter, or indicate it will not be a strong letter, you may need to circumvent the system by taking a few classes at another college to obtain the necessary letters.

Many schools have a central office that processes letters of recommendation, sometimes sending a summary letter representing the opinions of several instructors. If this is the case, it is important that you get your requests for letters of recommendation in as early as possible to assure that the extra processing does not delay your application.

How can you influence the quality of your letters of recommendation? Make a half-hour appointment to discuss career plans with the instructor from whom you have requested a recommendation. On the appointed day, dress in clothing appropriate for business. This will demonstrate the value you place on this meeting. Tell the individual your career choice, and ask his or her opinion of your selection. Make your request for a letter of recommendation. If you receive a favorable response, present the instructor with a packet containing a typed list of addresses of the medical schools to which you intend to apply, your curriculum vitae, personal statement, MCAT score or GPA (unless they are poor), and any other information you deem important. Include typewritten, stamped envelopes addressed to the schools to receive the letters. Provide a cover letter that includes the deadline for mailing the letters, a short summary of a few of your strong points, and how you can be reached to respond to questions, and a thank-you statement expressing your appreciation to the instructor for taking the time to write this letter. At the conclusion of your interview, ask if he or she has any questions, and be sure to thank the instructor for his or her time.

When you make your request, ask those writing recommendations if they are willing to write you a positive letter. All of the authors have heard stories from students not accepted that one of their recommendations was negative. One true story concerns a student who was at the top of her class and had outstanding MCAT scores. While in school, she became very close to one of her instructors, baby-sitting for his children, completing a major research project with him, and teaching his laboratory classes. The instructor agreed to write a letter for her and she did not question him regarding the type of letter he would write. Later, she was rejected from every medical school to which she applied. She eventually learned that she was rejected because this "friend" wrote a very negative letter. Apparently he felt that she was just too intelligent to "waste" her career in medicine, as he felt she should seek a Ph.D. Although it is difficult to know for sure if this situation could have been prevented, it illustrates the importance of always asking whether the individual is willing to write a favorable letter of recommendation.

When the schools have received your letters of recommendation, send thank-you notes to the instructors, as they write these letters every year and spend many hours doing so. Their time is valuable, so a thank-you letter two to three weeks after your request is appropriate. When you receive your acceptance into medical school, a personal visit to these professors and a second thank-you letter are strongly recommended.

Obtaining letters of recommendation is not a difficult task if you plan ahead. If you have worked hard in class and spent some time getting to know your professors, you will be rewarded.

C H A P T E R   1 4

CURRICULUM VITAE PREPARATION

"**Nothing is more terrible than activity without insight.**"

Thomas Carlyle

Preparing an up-to-date, professional-looking curriculum vitae, or résumé, should be done early in your career. It will be useful when you apply for jobs, scholarships, medical schools, and residencies. In addition, it will serve as a useful reference when you fill out forms, such as the American Medical College Application Service (AMCAS) application. Once you have learned what goes into a curriculum vitae, it will help you maintain an accurate outline of your accomplishments and pinpoint your deficiencies.

Curriculum vitaes differ in style; a variety of formats are acceptable. One style is exemplified in the sample curriculum vitae at the end of this chapter. A list of several books on résumés follows the chapter.

Placing a curriculum vitae on a computer disk has an advantage. As your career progresses, it can be quickly updated. When you need a special draft, professional printing companies can easily prepare a typeset version. However, photocopying your typed draft onto high-quality bond paper should prove sufficient for most uses.

Most résumés are divided into several sections. You may add and subtract areas as your credentials change and develop.

INTRODUCTION

The introductory section should include your name and your home and school addresses. Depending on the purpose of the résumé, you may want to provide a few brief statements concerning your professional goals.

EDUCATION

A section should be devoted to discussing your education to date, listing schools attended as well as majors and minors. Your grade point average should be included, especially if it is impressive. If you are presently in school, include your current status.

ACTIVITIES

Professional activities and social activities usually require separate sections, although they may be merged. If your college activities are minimal, you may want to include some of your major high school activities as well.

HONORS AND AWARDS

A list of all honors or awards received while in school should be provided. If you received an honor for only one year, do not list the year. For example, if you made the dean's list only one semester of your junior year, do not list the single year. Why advertise that your honor was limited? If you have not yet found a way to distinguish yourself, get to work!

PUBLICATIONS

If you have had an opportunity to publish a paper, definitely include it. As publication may take years to go to press, do not be afraid to include "Submitted," "In-progress," or "In-press."

PRESENTATIONS

Any demonstration of your speaking skills is important. If you have given a major lecture, include it, as employers and medical schools are particularly interested in your communication skills.

REFERENCES

Listing past and present employers and providing a means of contacting them is important to your résumé. A good employment record is something you should strive to maintain throughout your career. Rather than listing actual employers with their addresses, you may want to state, "References available upon request." Remember, if you list a reference, always ask the individual ahead of time so that you may be sure that he or she will provide a good recommendation.

As you progress through your years of college, you must take time out from studying. Medical schools look for "well-rounded" individuals who will make good physicians, as evidenced by participation in organized clubs and activities. Students who have not taken the time to interact with people but graduate at the top of their class may find it more difficult to secure a spot in medical school than they anticipated. Spending a great deal of time involved with friends does improve your social skills. Unfortunately, nonorganized activities such as partying are difficult to include on your curriculum vitae!

A variety of résumé styles are available and should be considered, depending on your individual credentials. A one-page résumé will suffice if you are in the early stages of your career. Brevity is an asset; do not write to take up space. The following curriculum vitae is provided as an example.

CURRICULUM VITAE

John Doe

ADDRESS: Box 242
                           Juniata, NE 68955
                           Phone 402-751-2670

PROFESSIONAL GOALS: Medical Doctorate
                           Residency: Pediatrics
                           Academic Medicine: Clinical practice
                              and research

EDUCATION TO DATE: College—University of Nebraska
                              Major—Communications
                              Minors—Biology and Philosophy
                              Grade Point Average 3.89 (4.00)
                           High School—Adams Central,
                              Juniata, Nebraska

PROFESSIONAL AND   Arts Council, Class Representative
SOCIAL ACTIVITIES: Phi Chi Phi Fraternity, Treasurer
                           Quad Council, Vice-president
                           Debate Team, Captain
                           Oratorical Society
                           Biology Club
                           University of NE Honors Program
                           University of NE Pep Band
                           Premedical Club, President
                           Intramural Sports: Volleyball and
                              Softball
                           Karate, Black Belt

HONORS AND AWARDS: Summa Cum Laude
                           Dean's List
                           Honors program (1 of 12 selected
                              from 1,200)
                           Sigma Gamma (Top 5% of Juniors)
                           Philosophy Student Essay Award

Debate Awards—1st place, State of
Nebraska; 6th Novice and 7th
Junior Varsity Nationals; 1st
LaCrosse; 2nd UNO and Iowa, 2nd
KSU; 4th KU; and 4th Yale

Speech Awards—Multiple in Oratory,
Impromptu, After Dinner, and
Demonstration

PUBLICATIONS:
PUBLISHED—

Doe, John: "Providing Medical Care
for the Homeless." *Nebraska Rag,*
Pp. 6–9, March 1989.

Wilson, J.J., and Doe, J.: "Alpha
Influence of Rat Liver Cell
Growth." *Biology Today* (In-press).

SUBMITTED—

Thomas, C.D., and Doe, J.: "Evidence
in Debate Rounds." *Forensics
Quarterly* (Submitted September 6,
1988).

PRESENTATIONS:

Alpha Receptor Activity and Cell
Growth. Department of Biology
Student Forum, January 18, 1989.

SPECIAL EDUCATION:

EMT-A, Licensed State of Nebraska
B.L.S. American Heart Association
A.L.S. American Swimming
Association

EMPLOYMENT:

Senior—Phlebotomist, Lincoln
General Hospital, 16 hours/week

Junior—Nurse's Aide, Thomas Home,
16 hours/week

Sophomore—EMT, Eastern
Ambulance, 8 hours/week

Freshman—Volunteer, South Hospital
Emergency Dept., 4 hours/week

References available upon request

BOOKS

Anthony, Rebecca and Roe, Gerald. *The Curriculum Vitae Handbook.* Rudi Publishing, 1998.

Bloch, Deborah P. *How to Write a Winning Resume.* Vgm Career Horizons, 1993.

Corwen, Leonard. *Your Resume: Key to a Better Job.* Arco, 1995.

Reed, Jean and Potter, Ray. *Resumes That Get Jobs.* 9th Edition, Arco, 1998.

Smith, Michael H. *The Resume Writer's Handbook.* Harper, 1995.

CHAPTER 15

WHERE TO APPLY

"Destiny is not a matter of chance, it is a matter of choice; it is not a thing to be waited for, it is a thing to be achieved."

William Jennings Bryan

Approximately one in two applicants fails to get into medical school. This result is often owing not to lack of ability, but to poor planning. Many students fail to make a realistic assessment of their chances of getting into individual medical schools and optimistically apply to only a few schools without analyzing their chances of being accepted into a particular program.

In one state medical school, for example, 90 percent of the accepted applicants are residents of the state. The other 10 percent are usually minority students or students with special qualifications, such as being related to an influential alumnus or patron. Yet each year several hundred people from other states apply to this state's medical school. Obviously their odds of gaining acceptance are very small.

Other students apply only to their state school. Although state schools may be inexpensive, applying to several other private institutions that accept applicants from all over the United States is a necessity for most students. Choosing private schools is an important process. Often students will disregard expensive private schools even though this may be their best opportunity for gaining acceptance. Some expensive private schools cater to students who may not meet the qualifications of public state schools. These students are forced to pay a premium to gain entrance. Although costly, most private schools offer financial aid to students. Attending private schools may entail incurring a large debt, but paying for medical school should not keep you from applying to these programs. If accepted to a private school and rejected by your own state school, you may now have a bargaining chip. You can always approach your state school director of admissions and ask, "Why am I accepted at this prestigious private school but not at my own state school, for which my parents have been paying taxes for years?" This argument may gain you a spot at your state school if you are willing to wait a year.

One option few students explore is to move to a state that offers less competition for medical school applicants. For example, in California and New York there are 10 to 20 applicants for every position, whereas in the Midwest that ratio may be as low as 1.5 to 1. Although it is usually difficult to become a resident of the more popular eastern and western states, gaining residency in the Midwest may take as little as six months. Before you make a move, be sure to check out the rules of each state regarding establishing residency. This information is usually available through the dean's office of state medical schools.

The best way to select medical schools is to review the Association of American Medical Colleges' book *Medical School Admissions Requirements*. Statistics are provided that help you choose schools based on the type of applicants each school selects. You should compare your credentials to the requirements of the schools you are considering. Some of the criteria you should consider include the following:

1. Percent of in- or out-of-state applicants selected

2. Admission class requirements

3. Average total and science GPA of accepted applicants

4. Average MCAT score of accepted applicants

5. Tuition (for private schools, usually the greater the cost, the easier to gain admission)

6. Special considerations (family ties, political ties, school affiliations, and minority status)

7. School location (Schools tend to favor applicants from the same geographical area.)

8. Success of previous applicants from your school (Your premedical advisor should have this data.)

9. Special qualifications (Some schools favor older applicants, applicants with advanced degrees, research-oriented applicants, applicants interested in rural practice, etc.)

10. Idiosyncracies (Several schools have atypical admission criteria that may be used to your advantage; e.g., one school no longer requires its applicants to take the MCAT.)

Once you have determined a list of schools that are most likely to accept you, check your list against the recommendations of your premedical advisor. He or she should know where students from your college have previously been accepted. Some medical schools are more apt to accept candidates from certain colleges because of their familiarity with the quality of applicants they have provided in the past. This may provide you with an important edge when being considered for admission.

Some states offer programs that provide special opportunities to attend certain public and private out-of-state schools. In particular, students from states that do not have medical schools should contact their premedical advisor to see if any special arrangements have been made to allow them special entrance status into certain schools.

Apply early! Send for applications to each school your junior year. Spend your summer evaluating programs and completing applications. Be sure to have the American Medical College Application Service (AMCAS) send your applications to each of the schools you are considering.

When looking into medical schools, be sure to consider schools that offer doctorate degrees in osteopathic medicine (D.O.). Although the philosophy is slightly different from that of medical doctorate schools, physicians who graduate from these schools take the same board exams and have equivalent practice opportunities. In addition, in some cases, it is slightly easier to obtain acceptance into these schools.

Selecting medical schools takes a great deal of thought. Evaluate every school you consider carefully. A realistic and objective determination of your chances of being accepted into a given medical school will increase your odds of being offered a medical school position.

PUBLICATIONS

Medical School Admission Requirements, 1999–2000. Association of American Medical Colleges, 1998.

ORGANIZATIONS

American Association of Colleges of Osteopathic Medicine Application Service, 6110 Executive Boulevard, Suite 405, Rockville, Maryland 20852-3991

American Medical College Application Service, Association of American Medical Colleges, 2501 M Street N.W., LBBY-26, Washington, D.C. 20037-1300

Director, WAMI Program, University of Washington (SC-64), School of Medicine, Seattle, Washington 98195

Office of Contract Services, New England Board of Higher Education, 45 Temple Place, Boston, Massachusetts 02111

Professional Student Exchange Program—Western Interstate Commission for Higher Education, P.O. Drawer P, Boulder, Colorado 80301-9752

Southern Regional Education Board, 529 Tenth Street, N.W., Atlanta, Georgia 30318-5790

CHAPTER 16

INTERVIEWS

Six Ways to Make People Like You

1. Become genuinely interested in other people.
2. Smile.
3. Remember that a person's name is to that person the sweetest and most important sound in any language.
4. Be a good listener. Encourage others to talk about themselves.
5. Talk in terms of the other person's interests.
6. Make the other person feel important—and do it sincerely.

Dale Carnegie

The first phase of preparing for medical school interviews encompasses your entire college career. Good interviewing skills are not innate. Like playing the piano or driving a car, they are skills that must be learned. Look for activities and classes that develop interviewing skills. Consider taking an introductory speech class during your freshman year or joining the speech team. As you progress in your training, consider a second speech course. Talk to a speech instructor who can recommend an appropriate course. Many schools offer a class specifically dedicated to interviewing skills.

If formal speech training is not an option, try to join a Toastmasters or Achieve Club. These two organizations are speaking groups. Each week their members meet to deliver speeches to each other. The format allows practice of a variety of speeches, such as informative, persuasive, and after-dinner addresses. Additionally, members are called on to give one- to two-minute extemporaneous speeches on a variety of subjects. The membership fees are low, and the training is excellent.

Prepare for medical school interviews by taking every opportunity to be interviewed. If you can apply for a job, political position, or scholarship that requires an interview, do so. Career days sponsored by major companies are good opportunities to develop interviewing skills. As a junior or senior, sign up to be interviewed. The experience you gain is worth the time and effort required even if you eventually decline a position you are offered.

The second phase of preparation should begin a few months before medical school interviews. Arrange with an instructor, close friend, or family member to have several "practice" interviews. After these practice sessions, contact a speech professor and arrange a mock interview. He or she may charge a small fee, but such a person's expertise may uncover mannerisms that will detract from your interview performance. The assistance provided will definitely enhance interviewing skills. Another option is to have mock interviews organized through a premedical club. "Seasoned" senior members can provide sample interview questions and perform helpful practice interviews.

Preparation when approaching individuals for mock interviews is important. Provide a list of questions, but tell the interviewers that any questions they want to ask are fair game. The scope of medical school interview questions is broad. Popular question categories include health issues, science, current events, and medical ethics. A favorite open-ended question is "Tell me about yourself."

Most interviewers are not concerned with your opinions. They are more concerned with your ability to communicate in an organized and logical manner. They are trying to determine whether you can communicate with future patients. Are you friendly? Do you listen carefully? Can you defend yourself? Do you believe what you are saying? Are you confident? Can you react quickly? Are you nervous? These are the skills and qualities the interviewer is assessing. Only by preparing will the ability and insight to appear calm and relaxed, to defend a position, and to state your opinions with confidence be apparent. Answering practice questions allows for development of these abilities.

An interviewer may ask a variety of questions. The following is a list of a few of the more common questions. Practice your responses, but also practice answering questions on topics with which you have limited familiarity. You must have the ability to adapt to the questions quickly and to answer in an organized and logical manner.

Sample Questions

1. Tell me about yourself.

2. Where did you grow up?

3. When did you first decide you wanted to become a doctor?

4. Do you have any family members who are physicians?

5. What kind of medicine would you like to practice?

6. Where do you think you will want to live?

7. What do you think of the government's involvement in health care?

8. Is free health care a right?

9. What do you think about abortion?

10. What do you think about euthanasia?

11. What do you think about organ donation from nonviable infants?

12. What are your hobbies?

13. What do you do in your free time?

14. What was your favorite class in undergraduate school?

15. If you had to change anything about your education, what would you change?

16. What do you think is your greatest strength?

17. What do you think is your biggest weakness?

18. How do you feel about working with dying patients?

19. How do you handle depression?

20. What is the single most exciting event in your life to date?

21. What was your biggest failure and how did you handle it?

22. What is the most difficult decision you have ever made?

23. Have you ever watched anyone die?

24. Have you ever worked in a hospital?

25. Why do you want to be a doctor?

26. If you do not get into medical school, what will you do?

27. Why should we select you?

28. What research have you done?

29. Why did you get a "C" in General Chemistry?

30. What leadership roles have you assumed?

31. What is your favorite book or author and why?

32. What do you do for fun?

33. If you were told you could not go to medical school, what would your second career choice be?

34. Are you married?

35. Do you have children?

36. Do you plan to have children?

37. How does your spouse feel about you going to medical school?

38. Do your parents want you to go to medical school?

39. What is the single biggest factor in your selecting medicine as a career?

40. Who was your favorite teacher and why?

41. Where do you see yourself in five years? Ten years? Twenty years?

42. How much money do you want to make each year?

43. If you were given a million dollars, what would you do with it?

44. What do you believe the American role should be in helping foreign governments?

45. How do you feel about national health insurance?

46. How do you feel about working for a health maintenance organization?

47. How do you feel about working with indigent patients?

48. Do you think you would enjoy living in a small town?

49. Do you have any family members in medicine?

50. What was your most embarrassing moment?

51. Why did you pick medicine over dentistry?

52. Tell me about your family.

53. What is the most stressful situation you have ever been in?

54. What do you consider a good income?

55. Do doctors make too much money?

56. Where else did you apply to medical school?

57. Why did you pick this medical school?

58. How will you finance your medical school education?

59. Have you been accepted to other medical schools?

60. What do you hate?

61. What is your understanding of a typical day for a physician?

62. What do you think is the United States government's biggest problem?

63. Given the power, how would you reduce the national debt?

64. What do you think of the job the President is doing?

65. How would you feel about working for the government?

66. How do you think medical malpractice could be reduced?

67. Do you know any attorneys you like?

68. How do you like the climate here?

69. What is your number one environmental concern?

70. What is the most beautiful picture you have ever seen?

71. Do you think medicine is becoming too impersonal with the advent of technology?

72. A patient has been waiting two hours to see you and is very upset. What would you say to calm the patient down?

73. You receive a malpractice claim against you in the mail. How do you react?

74. What is your favorite hobby?

75. What is your favorite sport?

76. How do you think managed care will influence your practice of medicine?

In addition to these questions, be prepared to answer others that are posed for their "shock value." Applicants have been asked such personal questions as "When was the last time you masturbated?" and "When was the last time you had sex?" One frequent request is "Tell me your favorite joke."

Female applicants should be prepared to deal with questions that have a chauvinistic tone, such as "Are you married?" "Do you plan to have any children?" "When?" "How will your husband deal with your being a doctor?" "Is he supportive?" "Medical students and doctors have the highest divorce rate in the United States. Are you sure being a physician is worth the risk?" "How do you plan to have time for your children?" and "What form of birth control do you use?"

Although personal questions may seem embarrassing to you, they are in some respects reasonable. As a doctor, you will often find yourself asking patients intimate questions and you must be comfortable in doing so. Similarly, in answering these interview questions, your responses need to be articulated without shyness or reserve.

One question the applicant must be ready to answer is "Do you have any questions?" Be prepared! You should have three or four intelligent questions concerning the medical school, the basic science curriculum, and clinical instruction. You might also ask a special interest question, such as "Do you have any affiliation with any foreign countries for clinical clerkships?" or "What research opportunities are available for medical students?" If you are really confident, one approach is to turn the tables on the interviewer with the question "I am looking at several medical schools and have narrowed my choices to two. Why should I pick your medical school over Harvard?"

Be aware of the variety of interview styles. Major interviewing styles include passive, combative, soothing, and agreeable. Whether these tactics are deliberately undertaken or are consistent with the interviewer's personality is irrelevant. The important thing is to remain calm and to control your emotions whatever the interview style. Remember: Do not overreact to what you cannot control.

A third phase of preparation should be familiarizing yourself with your own curriculum vitae. Review all the classes you have taken and reacquaint yourself with the basic topics covered in each course. If you have done any research, review the papers you have written and the basic literature involved with the topic. Do not assume that you will remember the details of research you did two to three years ago. Finally, if there is a weakness in your record, have a well-planned and logical explanation.

Phase four of preparing for the interview is to dress appropriately. Men should wear a conservative suit and a dress tie. The new sport jacket you purchased for a night on the town should be left in your closet. Women should look for a conservative suit or dress. Excessive jewelry should be avoided. Obviously, both males and females should be well groomed, with neatly trimmed hair and manicured fingernails. Women should avoid flashy clothes and excessive makeup; men, unkempt bushy beards. Any dress or style that deviates from the norm should be avoided. This is not the time for the "real you" when it comes to appearance.

Phase five is to be on your guard. Watch out for displaying overt signs of nervousness. Practice speaking in a forceful voice to project confidence. If you are asked to speak up, you're not appearing as confident as you should. A favorite interview tactic is to place objects within your reach such as paper clips or pens. Do not pick them up. Your hands should be in your lap. Do not cross your arms, because this projects disinterest. A trick is to ask the interviewee to open a nailed-down window. Some interviewers may challenge you with false information to test your reaction. For example, you may be asked, "Why is one of your letters of recommendation negative?" Such tactics are uncommon, although they have occurred. Books are available on subliminal signs and gestures to watch for and are listed at the conclusion of this chapter. Finally, be aware of the "unknown" interviewer. Some programs ask a medical student, secretary, or tour guide waiting in the hall to complete an evaluation. Do not be surprised at an extremely odd interview. Applicants often report interviewers spent their entire meeting looking out the window. It is not fair, but it happens.

After completing your interview, be sure to take a moment to write down the name or names of your interviewers. Note the subjects discussed and points of interest covered. When you get home, send a thank-you note to each interviewer as well as the dean of the medical school. You should mention some of the points you enjoyed about their school and some of your reasons for wanting to attend it. If you interviewed early in the season, consider sending a follow-up letter reconfirming your interest to the selection committee a few weeks before the selection deadline. Carefully edit any letter you send. There are countless horror stories about the poorly written thank-you letter passed around during an admission committee meeting, providing everyone with a good laugh but destroying that candidate's chances for admission.

The interview is the culmination of all your efforts. For many medical schools, it is one of the most important aspects of their evaluation of candidates. If you have prepared for this day throughout your college career, you will present yourself well. Remember: The prepared applicant will present him- or herself in the best possible light.

REFERENCES

Carnegie, Dale. *How to Win Friends and Influence People*. Pocket Books, 1994 Reissue Edition.

Carnegie, Dale. *Quick and Easy Ways to Effective Speaking*. Pocket Books, 1990 Reissue Edition.

Flesch, Rudolf. *How to Write, Speak, and Think More Effectively*. NAL, 1994 Reissue Edition.

McDonnell, Sharon. *You're Hired: Secrets to Successful Job Interviews*. Arco, 1995.

Molloy, John T. *John T. Molloy's New Dress for Success*. Warner Books, 1988.

Molloy, John T. *New Women's Dress for Success*, Warner Books, 1996.

Payne, Richard A. *How to Get a Better Job Quicker*. Taplinger, 1987.

CHAPTER 17

MEDICAL SCHOOL SELECTION AND FINANCIAL AID

"Isn't it fantastic? A person has risked himself and dared to become involved with experimenting with his own life, trusting himself. To do this, to experiment with your own life, is very exhilarating, full of joy, full of happiness, full of wonder, and yet, it is also frightening. Frightening because you are dealing with the unknown, and you are shaking complacency."

Leo Buscaglia

The days of impatiently searching the mailbox are over. You have made it! Some of you are fortunate. Sitting in front of you are not one, but several letters of acceptance.

If you carefully evaluated your applications, you ought to have a pretty good idea of the factors you should consider in making your final medical school selection. Most students consider such issues as location, prestige, student opinion, type of training, grading policy, housing, and cost.

SELECTION

Location

Where you go for a residency may determine where you will live for the rest of your career. Being trained in a particular part of the United States gives you knowledge of the "standard of care" for that community. You become familiar with the various specialists available and who are the best consultants. In selecting a medical school, location may be less of an important consideration, as you can always opt for a residency where you eventually want to live. However, as a medical student, you will become more familiar with the residency training available close to your home institution, and like it or not, you may find it easier to obtain a residency position in a competitive specialty in an area close to your medical school.

As medical school can be stressful, many students prefer to be close to their families. A quick trip home after a tough exam can relieve some of the anxiety medical students experience. Selecting a program in a pleasant environment can also have its advantages. Students who have the opportunity to spend a relaxing weekend on the beach may have a big advantage over those trapped in colder climates.

Prestige

Many students consider the reputation of the institution a primary reason to select a medical school. The top schools offer a number of possible advantages, the most important being the opportunity to be instructed by the best-known individuals in their field. Unfortunately, however, renowned instructors sometimes devote more time to research and are less apt to be interested in teaching.

A second possible advantage is that a well-known school's reputation could help you obtain a competitive residency position. This may or may not be true. Although most residencies consider the institution where you are trained to be a factor, they may also consider other, perhaps more important, criteria, including National Board scores, grades, class rank, research, letters of recommendation, clerkships completed, and junior-year evaluations.

The top schools also offer the chance to work with medical students who are often considered the top medical students in the United States. However, if you do decide on one of the more competitive schools and plan to select a specialty with a limited number of positions, such as ophthalmology, orthopedics, emergency medicine, or neurosurgery, you need to keep in mind that you must still be near the top of your class, no matter where you train. It is questionable whether someone in the middle of his class at Harvard, other things being equal, can obtain a residency in a competitive field over someone at the top of his class at the University of Oklahoma. The theory "It is easier to be a big fish in a small pond" may hold true.

The following anecdote illustrates an important point. Prior to selecting a medical school, one of the authors asked his family physician the question "Where should I go to medical school?" His doctor's response was "Do you know where I went to medical school? Internship? Residency?" "No, where?" "Johns Hopkins for medical school, Massachusetts General for internship, and the Mayo Clinic for Internal Medicine." He then added, "In thirty years of practice, do you know how many of my patients or consulting physicians asked me where I trained?" "How many?" "None!" His point is that you can get the most prestigious training you want, but much of your success will depend on your ability to deal with your patients and your fellow physicians. The exception is if you plan an academic career; the reputation of your training may be important throughout your academic career, since you will always be a product of "X."

Student Opinion

In selecting a school, contacting medical students should be a priority before making any decisions. If you are not acquainted with students at a prospective medical school, call the dean's office and ask the name and phone number of each class president. The cost of a few long-distance calls will be worth it in terms of getting the most out of your medical education. Topics covered should address issues discussed in this chapter.

Barron's Peterson, Princeton Review and REA all publish directories of medical schools in the United States. Any of these books, coupled with information in the Association of American Medical Colleges' *Medical School Admission Requirements,* should provide you with a fair idea of the type of training each school offers. A few final phone calls and a second visit to the schools in which you are interested should help you select the school that is best for you. Be thankful you have this decision to make, as many students are not so fortunate!

Types of Training

The first two years of courses differ little from school to school. The quality of lectures varies, however. It is important to contact medical students regarding the level and value of lectures in the first two years. There is a shortage of United States–born Ph.D.s in the basic sciences. Often you will have foreign lecturers who are difficult to understand. As medical schools tend to emphasize research above teaching, you should not be surprised to learn that most medical students will rank the quality of basic sciences lectures as "poor."

Of greater concern should be the variety of clinical training offered. Some schools specialize in providing excellent clinical training; others pride themselves as major research centers. In selecting a medical school, you must ask yourself which type of training is emphasized, clinical or research. A research center such as Harvard, Yale, UCLA, or Johns Hopkins may get your foot in the door early in your research career. However, as you progress, you will be judged more on your research accomplishments.

Some schools offer clinical training in hospitals for the indigent that provide a great deal of opportunity to see a lot and get hands-on experience. The disadvantage of this type of institution is the tendency to have students spend much of their clinic time doing "scut work," such as drawing blood and pushing patients to radiology, with less time devoted to actual instruction. If you are the type of person that learns by doing, this may be the school you should select.

Other schools emphasize a lecture approach combined with patient contact during your clinical years. Achieving an appropriate balance can be difficult. Often these schools are affiliated with private hospitals where patient contact is usually severely limited. As private patients do not like students practicing on them, expect to spend a significant amount of your clinical time observing.

As you select a medical school, perhaps the best advice is to look for balance. Many schools are affiliated with a university hospital, a private hospital, an inner-city hospital, and a veterans' hospital. The combination should give you the opportunity to discover what type of clinical training is most appropriate for you and the medical career you have chosen.

Grading Policy

Variety exists in the grading policy used by medical schools. Some offer a pass-fail system; others use the traditional letter grades. The concept of pass-fail was originally devised to decrease competition and stress for medical students. Unfortunately, residency programs want a means of evaluating students; therefore most schools have ways of ranking students regardless of the system. Selecting a school based on "less competition" may be an error.

Looking at the attrition (failure) rate of a medical school may be more important. No more than 5 percent of a class fails to complete the training in most medical schools. Higher percentages should be questioned.

Housing

As you consider medical schools, evaluating your living conditions will be an issue. Students who select schools in large cities will often be forced to incur higher debt not only for tuition, but for living expenses as well. In some instances, the cost of renting an apartment may actually approach or exceed your medical school tuition. Depending on the area you select, your options regarding living quarters will vary considerably.

Some medical schools offer student housing. This is often an inexpensive apartment complex offering the advantage of close proximity to your medical institution. As most of the students you live near will be in medical training, it provides you with an excellent opportunity to interact with classmates, nursing students, residents, and students in the allied health fields.

A few medical schools are affiliated with medical fraternities. This usually involves living in a large, old mansion or an apartment complex. Meals are often eaten as a group. Not only does this provide inexpensive room and board, it offers a pleasant environment with opportunities to interact and socialize with your classmates.

Many students choose to live in apartments or rent homes away from their medical center. This allows living near people who are not caught up in the daily grind of medical school. This break into reality may be a pleasant relief from the stress of being at or near a medical school campus.

You will spend four years in medical school. Some students consider purchasing a home. Often an older three- to four-bedroom home can be purchased at a reasonable price in the vicinity of your medical school. If you are a first-time home buyer with little or no income, you may qualify for reduced government loans with low interest rates. Rooms can be rented out to classmates to cover mortgage payments, taxes, and maintenance costs. The home can be inexpensively furnished in "Early American

Salvation Army" for as little as $1,000, which is tax deductible. If you manage your property carefully, you may generate extra cash for your education or, at the very least, to live in your home for free. At the completion of your training, you can often sell the home at a profit to a freshman medical student, especially if the buyer can assume your low-interest loan and you can demonstrate how you lived in the home "free" while you completed your medical training.

Cost

Unless your parents are wealthy and have offered to pay for your medical education, cost should be a consideration in your list of factors in selecting a medical school. If you received acceptance only at an expensive private school, you may be obligated to incur a large financial debt. If you have an opportunity to attend an inexpensive state school, you should give this institution serious thought. Total four-year costs at private schools can be as high as $150,000, whereas public school costs can be as low as $30,000. When you start to look at repayment schedules of $1,000 a month for 20 years, you may decide that cheaper is better.

Financial Aid

Finances should never prevent anyone from attending medical school! Finding the funds to finance your medical education may prove difficult, but it is not impossible. A number of scholarships, grants, and loans are available from many sources.

Scholarships for gifted students are available. These funds are given to students without any expectation of repayment. Scholarships should be applied for immediately after acceptance to a particular medical school, as applications often must be in early for consideration.

Some medical schools have scholarships, grants, or loans available to students willing to follow up their medical career with a practice in a rural community. The time commitment may be 5 to 10 years, but this may offer a reasonable mechanism for financing medical school.

Although increasingly hard to come by, each branch of the United States military offers full-tuition scholarships. These have the advantage of paying the entire tuition as well as providing living expenses. Payback periods are usually four years of military service after completing residency requirements.

Most medical students utilize one or more of the federal government student loan programs. A variety of loans are available. Most are based on the student's financial background and that of his or her parents.

The following provides a brief overview of public and private programs available. Contact the financial aid office of the medical school you plan to attend for up-to-date information.

Air Force, Army, Navy, and National Guard: Not need-based. Provides full tuition, living stipend, supplies, and book allowance. Obligates recipient to one year of military service for each year of financial support.

American Association of University Women (AU):   Not need-based. For information, write to AU Educational Foundation Programs, 2410 Virginia Avenue, N.W., Washington, D.C. 20037.

American Medical Women's Association, Medical Education Loan Program: Women in their first, second, or third year of medical school are eligible to apply. Applicants must be U.S. citizens or permanent residents attending a U.S. institution full-time and be student members of AMWA. For information, write to American Medical Women's Association, Medical Education Loan Program, 801 North Fairfax Street, Suite 400, Alexandria, Virginia 22314.

Business and Professional Women's Foundation Scholarship Program: Need-based. The program assists women 30 and older to seek the education necessary for entry into or advancement within the work force. Applicants must be within 24 months of completing an accredited program at a U.S. institution. Applications are available only from October 1 to April 1. The deadline is April 15. For information, write to Business and Professional Women's Foundation Scholarship Program, 2012 Massachusetts Avenue, N.W., Washington, D.C. 20036.

Clairol Loving Care Scholarships: Need- and merit-based. Open to women at least 30 years old in their final two years of medical studies. For information, write to Scholarships, BPW Foundation, 2012 Massachusetts Avenue, N.W., Washington, D.C. 20036.

Exceptional Financial Need Scholarship (EFN):   Need-based. Students must be from a severely disadvantaged background. Scholarship grant covers tuition, books, and fees annually with no repayment expected. Must commit to practice of Primary Care Medicine or General Dentistry upon graduation.

Federal Subsidized Stafford Student Loan (FSSL): Need-based. Borrow up to $8,500 per year, maximum $65,500. Variable interest rate not to exceed 8.25 percent. Repayment begins six months after you graduate, leave school, or drop below half-time enrollment.

Federal Unsubsidized Stafford Loan (FUSSL): Not need-based. Borrow up to $10,000 per year, maximum $73,000. Variable interest rate not to exceed 8.25 percent. Repayment schedule is variable.

Fellowships for Native Americans: Need-based. Students must be at least one-fourth American Indian, Eskimo, Aleut, or a member of a tribe recognized by the Bureau of Indian Affairs and in financial need. For information, write to American Indian Scholarship, Inc., 5106 Grand Avenue, N.E., Albuquerque, New Mexico 87108.

Financial Assistance for Disadvantaged Health Professions Students (FADHPS): Need-based. Students must be from a severely disadvantaged background. Scholarship grant covers tuition, books, and fees annually with no repayment expected.

Perkins Loan: Need-based. Borrow up to $5,000 per year, maximum $30,000. Interest rate 5 percent. Repayment begins nine months after you graduate, leave school, or drop below half-time enrollment.

A number of options are available to finance your medical education. For students willing to incur a debt, the federal government provides a variety of financing mechanisms. Private companies may lend money to medical students, but the interest rates can be high. A number of references follow this chapter. For expert help, contact the financial aid office of the medical schools you are considering.

Selecting a medical school is a challenge. Finances should not stand in your way of attending medical school! Your decision involves consideration of location, perceived quality of education, opinions of students, and financial considerations. Take the time to consider all of the information available before making your final decision.

PUBLICATIONS

Career Choices: Health Professions Opportunities for Minorities. Free. Office of Statewide Health Planning and Development, Health Professions Career Opportunity Program, 1600 Ninth Street, Room 441, Sacramento, California 95814.

Educational Survival Skills Reading Package. Free. Office of Statewide Health Planning and Development, Health Professions Career Opportunity Program, 1600 Ninth Street, Sacramento, California 95814.

Financial Advice for Minority Students Seeking an Education in the Health Professions. Free. Office of Statewide Health Planning and Development, Health Professions Career Opportunity Program, 1600 Ninth Street, Room 441, Sacramento, California 95814.

Financial Aid for Minorities in Health Fields. Garrett Park Press, P.O. Box 190, Garrett Park, Maryland 20896.

Financial Planning and Management Manual for U.S. Medical Students. Association of American Medical Colleges. Publication Orders, AAMC, 2450 N Street N.W., Washington, D.C. 20037-1127

Financial Planning Guide for Medical Students in the U.S. Educational and Scientific Trust of Pennsylvania Medical Society, 20 Erford Road, Lemoyne, Pennsylvania 17043.

Haller, E.H., and Myers, R.A. (Eds.), *Searching, Teaching, Healing: American Indians and Alaskan Natives in Biomedical Research Careers.* $9.95. Futura Publishing Company, Inc., 295 Main Street, P.O. Box 330, Mount Kisco, New York 10549.

Health Pathways. Free. Office of Statewide Health Planning and Development, Health Professions Career Opportunity Program, 1600 Ninth Street, Room 441, Sacramento, California 95814.

Informed Decision-Making: Part I, Financial Planning and Management for Medical Students; Part II, Sources of Financial Assistance for Medical School. National Medical Fellowships,

Inc. 1990. 254 West 31st Street, New York, New York 10001.

Minorities in Medicine: A Guide for Premedical Students. Free. Office of Statewide Health Planning and Development, Health Professions Career Opportunity Program, 1600 Ninth Street, Room 441, Sacramento, California 95814.

Schlachter, G.A., *Directory of Financial Aids for Women.* A list of over 1,600 scholarships, fellowships, loans, grants, internships, awards, and prizes available to women. Also includes a list of state sources of educational benefits and a bibliography of financial aid directories. Reference Service Press, 1100 Industrial Road, Suite 9, San Carlos, California 94070.

Schlachter, G.A., and Goldstein, S.E, *Directory of Financial Aids for Minorities.* Includes over 2,000 scholarships, fellowships, loans, grants, awards, and internships for African American, Hispanic, Asian, and Native American sudents. Reference Service Press, 1100 Industrial Road, Suite 9, San Carlos, California 94070.

The Student Guide: Five Federal Financial Aid Programs. Department of Education. Federal Student Aid Information Center, P.O. Box 84, Washington, D.C. 20044.

ORGANIZATIONS AND PROGRAMS

AAMC MEDLOANS Program, Section for Student Services, Association of American Medical Colleges, 2450 N Street N.W., Washington, D.C. 20037-1127

Air Force, USAF Health Professions Recruiting, Airman Memorial Bldg., 5211 Auth Road, Suite 201, Suitland, MD 20746.

Army, AMEDD Regional Director, Bldg. 1, Suite A, Walter Reed Army Medical Center, Washington, D.C. 20307.

Bureau of Indian Affairs Higher Education Grant Program, Postsecondary Education, 18th and C Streets, N.W., Washington, D.C. 20204.

National Health Service Corps Scholarship Program, Bureau of Health Care Delivery and Assistance, Room 7-16, Parklawn Building, 5600 Fishers Lane, Rockville, Maryland 20857.

Navy, Navy Recruiting District, Suite 301, Naval Belcrest Road, Hyattsville, Maryland 20782.

Scholarship Program for Minority Students, National Medical Fellowships, Inc., Room 1820, 250 W. 57th St., New York, New York 10107.

CHAPTER 18

SPECIAL APPLICANTS: MINORITIES, OLDER STUDENTS, AND WOMEN

**"We Rarely Gain A Higher or Larger View
Except When It Is Forced Upon Us Through
Struggles Which We Would Avoid If We Could"**

Charles Cooney

Providing a perspective on special medical school applicants is difficult. Placing a variety of individuals into "special" status makes generalizations difficult. What is unique about a certain individual may be either appealing or repellent to a particular medical school and consequently make that individual's acceptance much easier or harder, depending on the circumstances involved. This chapter makes a few observations, provides an overview of the data available, and offers some suggestions. No information provided is absolute. What is true for one individual may be completely irrelevant for another.

MINORITIES

U.S. citizens who are African Americans, Puerto Ricans, Native Americans, Mexican Americans, and individuals from low-income families will generally find acceptance into medical school easier with other variables being equal. Unfortunately, although the doors to medical school may be open, the exit, diploma in hand, is statistically more difficult.

During the MCAT you will have the opportunity to take advantage of the Association of American Medical Colleges Medical Minority Applicant Registry (Med-MAR). The Med-MAR circulates information concerning your biographical background to the admissions offices of various medical schools. If a particular school is interested, they will contact you directly regarding your application. Further information concerning this program can be obtained by writing to the Minority Student Clearinghouse, Association of American Medical Colleges, 2450 N Street, N.W., Washington, D.C. 20037.

Most medical schools are seeking to increase minority enrollment. The problem is, if you have a poor academic background, few medical schools provide the supplemental training necessary to complete tough medical school courses. With the massive amount of material that must be covered to complete a medical school education, little time is available to make up for deficiencies in preparation. If you consider yourself to be academically marginal, strongly consider taking extra steps to assure that you will be able to complete medical school.

Most students find the first two years of basic sciences the biggest challenge of their medical school education. If your science background is weak or deficient, consider adopting one of the following courses:

1. Ask to have your admission deferred for one year. During this time, take extra undergraduate course work in anatomy, physiology, embryology, histology, biochemistry, and microbiology. Since you have already been accepted to medical school, grades received are irrelevant. By expanding your science background in these courses, you will make the successful completion of the basic science portion of medical school significantly easier.

2. If you are unwilling to take a year off or are unable to obtain a deferment, consider taking gross anatomy or biochemistry at a medical school the summer before your freshman year. Across the nation, several medical schools offer these courses. All medical schools provide a list of summer courses available. Often they can be audited at no charge. Although it will not be a fun summer, you will have the jump on one of your most difficult freshman courses.

   As an alternative to taking a single summer course, some medical schools offer summer "prep" courses for minority students. Often these are "cram" courses that review key concepts in several freshman classes. A current list of summer enrichment programs may be obtained by writing to the Minority Student Information Clearinghouse, AAMC, Suite 200, One Dupont Circle, N.W., Washington, D.C. 20036.

3. Call the Dean of Minority Affairs prior to accepting a position in the medical school you are considering. This person's name and number may be obtained by contacting the dean's office of the medical school or by consulting the *Medical School Admissions Requirements* handbook published by the Association of American Medical Colleges. Ask how minority students with your background have done in the past. In particular, ask what percentage of minority students completed their medical education and what programs are available to assist students with academic difficulties. If minority students do not fare well, what programs does the school offer for increasing the odds of successfully completing training? Find out if the basic sciences can be extended from two to three years. Ask what happens to a student who flunks one, two, or three freshman courses. Can the first and second years be repeated? Although these are tough questions to ask, it is better to know before problems arise. Be aware that in some schools, if you don't pass every single class, you're automatically *out*!

Your financial status may be a concern when applying to medical schools. Because of the variety of financial assistance available for public and private medical schools, do not think you are unqualified to apply to a school because of your financial background. Most schools have financial aid directors to assist you in securing the grants and loans necessary to complete your medical school education. For a more complete discussion, see Chapter 17 and the references provided.

OLDER APPLICANTS

More and more older individuals are applying to medical school. Few studies are available revealing the problems older applicants face. Although the percentage of older applicants accepted is slowly growing, statistics demonstrate that as age increases, the chances of being accepted into medical school decrease. According to data from the American Medical Association, the percentages of men and women matriculating into medical school, broken down by age groups, are as follows: 78 percent of men and 73 percent of women, ages 21–23; 44 percent of men and 43 percent of women, ages 24–27; 40 percent of men and 53 percent of women, ages 28–31; 42 percent of men and 51 percent of women, ages 32–34; 41 percent of men and 46 percent of women, ages 35–37; and 27 percent of men and 34 percent of women, ages 38 and over.

As difficulty in gaining admission increases with age, older applicants should strive to demonstrate what their unique qualities will contribute to a medical school class and their future role as physicians. Many older applicants have pursued interests in unrelated fields and late in life decide to follow careers in medicine. It is important to demonstrate to admissions committees that you still have what it takes to be a successful medical student. This may mean retaking basic science courses like general biology, inorganic and organic chemistry, and physics. As it has probably been a long time since you took a standardized test, it is important that preparation for the MCAT begin long before the exam and that you make a serious effort to score well the first time you take the test. If you had mediocre grades many years ago as a college student, it is even more important for you to excel in the courses you take prior to applying to medical school. The fact that you are now older and more mature will be considered by admissions committees, but you must demonstrate proficiency in science courses if you want to be accepted.

Medical committees may be concerned about the disruption medical school can present to your family. It is important that you be able to discuss your motivations for seeking medical school entrance late in life, to show that you are adequately prepared to meet the emotional and financial responsibilities of returning to school. If you are not currently involved in a health care profession, it may be wise to consider seeking part-time employment in a medical setting before completing your application. Do everything you can to demonstrate that the major change in your career plans is well thought out and completely rational.

WOMEN

The discussion of women as special applicants is almost unnecessary. Discrimination based on sex, at least in regard to medical school acceptance, is minimal to nonexistent. Medical schools now realize that women make excellent physicians. Studies demonstrate that women perform as well as and sometimes better than their male counterparts. Since the 1950s, the percentage of women accepted into medical school has been increasing. In the 1991–92 classes, of 13,700 female applicants, 6,433, or 46.9

percent, were accepted. This compares to 19,601 male applicants with 10,493 accepted, or 53.5 percent.

As was discussed in Chapter 16, female applicants should expect to be queried on such issues as personal relationships, effect of medical training on childbearing, and spouse support. It is not illegal to ask these questions, but it is illegal to base decisions of acceptance to medical school on the answers given.

In studies evaluating premedical student performance, men had slightly higher science GPAs and women had slightly higher overall GPAs. Men scored slightly higher in all areas of the MCAT except reading. In a 1987 American Association of Medical Colleges study of matriculating students, women showed a lower level of parental support and lower parental incomes. Women also had a higher debt at the completion of medical school. In medical school clerkships, women scored similarly to men except in obstetrics/gynecology and patient interviewing courses, in which women outscored men. Studies have shown that women suffer higher levels of anxiety and depression during medical school. They also experience greater sexism from faculty and staff. In spite of this, they perform at equal levels to male medical students.

Women tend to have a greater commitment to primary care specialties than men. They also tend to select pediatrics, ob/gyn, psychiatry, and pathology. Women are not as active in surgical specialties.

PUBLICATIONS

American Medical Association's Department of Women in Medicine. *In the Marketplace: Work Patterns, Practice Characteristics and Incomes of Women Physicians.* 1987. Free. American Medical Association, 515 North State Street, Chicago, Illinois 60610; 312-464-4392.

American Medical Association's Department of Women in Medicine. *The Residency Interview: A Guide for Medical Students.* 1986. Free. American Medical Association, 515 North State Street, Chicago, Illinois 60610; 312-464-4392.

Arnold, R., et al. "Taking Care of Patients—Does It Matter Whether the Physician Is a Woman?" *Western Journal of Medicine,* 149:729–733, December 1988.

Bickel, J., *Medicine and Parenting: A Resource for Medical Students, Residents, Faculty and Program Directors.* Washington D.C.: AAMC, 1991. (Call 202-828-0416 to order.)

Bickel, M.A., "Women in Medical Education." *New England Journal of Medicine,* 319:1579–1584, December 15, 1988.

Bowman, M., and Allen, D., *Stress and Women Physicians,* second edition. New York: Springer-Verlag Publishers, 1990.

"Careers of Woman Physicians: Choices and Constraints" and "Taking Care of Patients—Does It Matter Whether the Physician Is a Woman?" *Western Journal of Medicine,* December 1988, 149 (6). California Medical Association, 44 Gough Street, San Francisco, California 94103.

Epps, A.C., et al. *MED REP at Tulane: Effectiveness of a Medical Education Reinforcement and Enrichment Program for Minorities in the Health Professions,* 1985. Futura Publishing Company, Inc., 295 Main Street, P.O. Box 330, Mount Kisco, New York 10549.

Grant, L., "The Gender Climate of Medical School: Perspectives of Women and Men Students." *Journal of the American Medical Women's Association,* 43:109–119, July/August 1988.

A Handbook for Minority Pre-Med Students. 1987. American Medical Student Association, 1890 Preston White Drive, Reston, Virginia 22091.

Helping Hands: Horizons Unlimited In Medicine, Order No. OP-160. Order Department, American Medical Association, P.O. Box 10946, Chicago, Illinois 60610.

Higgins, E.J., *Participation of Women and Minorities on U.S. Medical School Faculties.* Association of American Medical Colleges, 1985.

Kaplan, S., "Motivations of Women Over 30 for Going to Medical School." *Journal of Medical Education,* 56:856–857, 1981.

Medical School Admissions Requirements, 1998. Association of American Medical Colleges, 2450 N Street N.W., Washington, D.C. 20037-1127

Minorities and Women in the Health Fields. U.S. Department of Health and Human Services, DHHS Pub. No. (HRSA) HRS-DV 84-5, September 1986.

Minority Student Opportunities in United States Medical Schools.
1986. Association of American Medical Colleges. Publication
Orders, Association of American Medical Colleges, 2450 N Street
N.W., Washington, D.C. 20037-1127

Minority Students in Medical Education Facts and Figures.
Association of American Medical Colleges Section of Minority
Affairs, March 1988, 2450 N Street N.W., Washington, D.C.
20037-1127

Prieto, D.O., et al., *Simulated Minority Admissions Exercise.*
Association of American Medical Colleges, 1986.

PROGRAM

Health Pathways. Office of Statewide Health Planning and
Development, HPCOP Program, Room 441, 1600 9th Street,
Sacramento, California 95814.

CHAPTER 19

WHAT TO DO IF YOU DO NOT GET IN

1832 Lost Job

1832 Defeated for Legislature

1833 Failed in Business

1834 Elected to Legislature

1835 Sweetheart Died

1836 Had a Nervous Breakdown

1838 Defeated for Speaker

1844 Defeated for Nomination to Congress

1846 Elected to Congress

1848 Lost Re-election

1849 Rejected for Land Officer

1856 Defeated for Nomination for Vice-President

1858 Defeated for Senate

1860 **ELECTED PRESIDENT OF THE UNITED STATES**

Abraham Lincoln

What do you do if you are not accepted to medical school? Even though the applicant pool is declining, almost one-half of all students applying to medical school are faced with this question every year. Few applicants consider this a possibility, and thus most do not have contingency plans. Those who do find something else often do so in a rash manner, leading to poor decisions that actually make future acceptance into medical school even more difficult. Several options are available, each with significant advantages and disadvantages. Only after evaluating all the alternatives should a decision be made.

Be realistic and plan for the possibility of rejection. Knowing you have other choices will decrease the mental anguish. Remain confident that you will eventually be selected. The declining applicant pool will work in your favor.

An important question to ask yourself is "Why wasn't I selected?" It may have been your grade point average, MCAT scores, bad interviews, poor letters of recommendation, missed deadlines, late applications, too few applications sent, incomplete applications, inappropriate school selection, or any combination of the above. You must address the problem honestly. More than likely, you will be able to determine your areas of weakness. If not, contact your premedical advisor, who may be able to give you ideas on areas that need improvement. If necessary, contact the dean or director of admissions of the medical schools to which you applied. Usually vague reasons are given for applicant rejection. However, they may be able to give you a few specific ideas for improving your application credentials.

IMPROVING MCAT SCORES

If your MCAT scores are below the national average, take a review course or buy several review books. Go all out in preparing for your second exam. Allow enough time in your schedule so you can confidently say that you did the best you could. Many individuals who take a review course or study review books do not devote the time necessary to receive full benefit. For example, review courses often consist of several weeks of lectures and exams, as well as outside work. Due to time constraints, students often do not complete all the work. This extra preparation may make a difference in MCAT scores.

You must make an effort to cover all the bases. If a careful analysis of your academic record reveals your MCAT score to be a primary deficit, also look toward improving your second weakest area. For example, a possibility is to take additional science courses or find a part-time job in a health care setting. Always do more than necessary. Even though a dean says your MCAT scores are low, other deficiencies are likely to exist as well.

GETTING NEW LETTERS OF RECOMMENDATION

When reapplying to medical school it is a good idea to ask different individuals for letters of recommendation. Students are often unaware that the professor they thought really liked them may have described them as "poor applicants" for medical school. Taking a few additional science courses from new instructors to obtain different letters of recommendation may significantly change your application as well as increase your grade point average. Take every reasonable measure to improve your application.

TAKING EXTRA COURSE WORK / IMPROVING GRADE POINT AVERAGE

If your science GPA is marginal, consider taking additional upper-division undergraduate or graduate science courses. Prior to your reapplication, you may be able to complete two summer school courses and several fall semester classes. If a medical school is near your residence, consider taking one or two classes there. This gives you an opportunity to demonstrate to admissions committees that you can handle more difficult science or medical school courses.

As an undergraduate student taking graduate courses, you should have considerable leeway in selecting classes. For example, you could take classes like gross anatomy, biochemistry, embryology, neuroanatomy, or histology. These classes will take a great deal of study time, especially if you are doing "A" work! As you are not an official graduate student, you have an advantage. First, you are not locked into a two- to three-year graduate program. Second, you can be selective regarding the courses you choose. For example, if your local medical school's biochemistry course is well taught, you can take it instead of one not so well presented. If you were not a science major in undergraduate school, you should slowly ease yourself into graduate science classes. Suddenly taking 16 hours of graduate medical science courses could overwhelm you, leading to irreparable damage to your previous GPA and eliminating your chances of getting into medical school.

CHANGING RESIDENCE

Consider your state of residence when rejected. If you live on the East or West Coast, it is much more difficult to get into medical school. For your fifth year of undergraduate work, you might consider moving to a less crowded and less competitive Midwestern state for additional course work. Establishing a new state of residence gives you another chance to gain acceptance into a less competitive state medical school. Before you embark on such a change, be sure to contact the public medical schools of the states you are considering to determine how state residency requirements are met. They vary from state to state, and some are more easily fulfilled than others.

REAPPLYING

In making your initial decision, you may have overestimated your chances of acceptance into some of the top medical schools. If so, you may need to set your sights a little lower and apply to more private schools or consider a Doctorate in Osteopathic Medicine (D.O.). D.O. schools offer training similar to Medical Doctorate (M.D.) schools and at the completion of training, D.O.s have the same responsibility and license to practice as M.D.s. These schools are slightly less well known than most American Medical Association Medical Doctorate schools, and as a result, competition is somewhat less intense.

If you were given a waiting list position or granted interviews at some medical schools, it is a good idea to reapply to these programs. If you were selected for an interview the first time, improvements in your second application may increase your odds of acceptance. Applications should be sent early. Remember, the odds of acceptance decrease at many schools as the final deadline approaches. Many schools fill positions as the applications arrive. Consequently, as the number of spots decreases, the level of competition for the remaining seats increases.

POST-BACCALAUREATE PROGRAMS

Few students are aware that a number of undergraduate institutions offer post-baccalaureate programs for students interested in medical school. Some applicants to these programs are students who had previous careers in non-health-related fields and are returning to college for a one-year concentrated program in inorganic and organic chemistry, biology, and physics. Most of these programs are affiliated with a medical school, and their graduates are often given preference for admission to the associated medical school. Many of these programs are geared toward minority students previously rejected by medical schools; they sometimes, however, accept other students who show academic promise. Your premedical advisor should be able to provide you with an up-to-date list of post-baccalaureate programs. Currently available programs are listed at the conclusion of this chapter.

GRADUATE SCHOOL

A common choice for unsuccessful medical school applicants is graduate school. Rejected students often apply to medical-school-based graduate programs that provide convenient access to medical school courses and instructors. The advantage of these programs is that if a graduate program in anatomy is selected, part of your first year of medical school can often be waived at a future date. However, graduate schools in microbiology, pathology, physiology, pharmacology, and biochemistry may not provide such a practical choice. These programs offer completion of only one to two medical school courses, requiring you to start from scratch when you reapply to medical school.

A potential disadvantage of entering any graduate program is that you usually must finish the program prior to acceptance into medical school. This means two to three years of graduate school before you will be able to start on your desired career. Graduate school is not fun or easy. In many respects, it is more difficult than medical school. Graduate students are expected to maintain at least a "B" average. These "B's" must be maintained by completing difficult graduate classes, sometimes in direct competition with medical and dental students. In addition to course work, there is a graduate research project to complete. When you finish graduate school, you may or may not have raised your science grade point average. As a medical school applicant, you are competing against a large pool of graduate students that have done equally well or better in their graduate courses. Some have completed Ph.D.s, which may make them even more competitive. Another problem with graduate school is that it is difficult to excel at something you do not enjoy. You will be expected to spend hundreds of hours doing research on days, evenings, and weekends. It takes true dedication to complete this arduous program.

If you really enjoy research, graduate school may be a good option. Before you take the plunge, be aware of the ramifications graduate school presents. One final problem with graduate school is that if you do not do well, you may have sealed your fate, as your chances of being accepted into a medical school in the future decline dramatically.

FOREIGN MEDICAL SCHOOLS

Some premedical students consider a foreign medical education as an acceptable option. If this is your choice, be wary. United States–born citizens attending foreign medical schools often have problems with finances and the language barrier. Deficits found in foreign programs include poor faculty and equipment, mediocre curricula, and inadequate clinical training. Fewer than half of the U.S. citizens attending foreign medical schools eventually practice medicine in the United States. In addition, securing a residency in the United States is even more difficult. In many cases you may be effectively excluded from the more competitive residencies, such as surgery, orthopedics, emergency medicine, ophthalmology, and radiology.

Should you still decide this is your best option, there are a number of foreign medical schools to consider. Only students enrolled in foreign medical schools listed in the World Directory of Medical Schools, published by the World Health Organization, are eligible either to transfer to a United States medical school or to practice in the United States upon passing the Foreign Medical Graduate Examination in the Medical Sciences. A copy can be obtained by contacting the United Nations Bookshop.

A number of articles and studies have been done evaluating foreign medical schools and foreign-trained doctors. A few are referenced at the end of this chapter. If you are interested in a foreign medical school, be sure to contact graduates of the program. Find out how many students each year either successfully matriculate into a U.S. medical school or are accepted into U.S. residency programs. Clinical training is often the major weakness of foreign schools. Find out where the clinical years are spent. You should also find out whether the school allows transfer into a U.S. medical school after completion of the basic science portion of your training.

Another option for the foreign medical school graduate is to apply to a Fifth Pathway program in the United States after completing foreign medical school, but prior to receiving the medical degree. This is essentially a fifth year of clinics spent in an American Medical Association–approved clinical clerkship program. Successful completion allows the student to apply to a U.S. internship or residency after successfully passing the Federation Licensing Examination. You can write to the American Medical Association for a list of possible programs.

One final problem with foreign medical schools is the difficulty in obtaining student loans. A 1986 amendment to the Higher Education Act limits federally funded guaranteed student loans to U.S. citizens studying in foreign medical schools. Few foreign medical schools meet the eligibility requirements. To be eligible, 60 percent of the medical school's enrollment must consist of natives of the country in which the school is located, or at least 50 percent of the U.S. citizen graduates in the previous two years must have passed the FMGEMS. Although many U.S. citizens choose a foreign medical school as a route to obtaining the M.D., the potential for disappointment is great.

ALTERNATIVES TO MEDICAL DOCTORATES

An option few rejected medical applicants consider is a one- to two-year program in a related medical field. Programs in medical technology, respiratory therapy, occupational therapy, speech therapy, physical therapy, paramedics, or accelerated nursing should be considered. If you do well, this offers you a means to work part-time during medical school, teaches you a significant amount of practical clinical medicine, and demonstrates your commitment to the health field. Since it is health care related, you may have more enthusiasm for your training than you might have had in a graduate science program.

If you decide to drop medicine as your primary goal, there are many fields to consider. If you are interested in research, a Ph.D. may be possible in such areas as biochemistry, physiology, experimental psychiatry, anatomy, biology, microbiology, or the life sciences. If you are primarily interested in working with people, positions in counseling, clinical psychology, personnel management, or teaching may be of interest. Should you want to be involved in a medically related profession, careers in dentistry, optometry, podiatry, nursing, occupational therapy, physical therapy, pharmacy, radiation physics, medical technology, physician's assistance, or hospital administration may be appropriate. If income or prestige is a primary concern, careers in law, engineering, or business can provide interesting possibilities.

Rejection from medical school is a discouraging event in any student's life. Overcoming that rejection is difficult. Do not take it as a reflection on your suitability as a doctor. No study has ever been able to demonstrate a strong correlation between undergraduate grades or MCAT scores and eventual performance as a physician. Numerous people have received one or more rejections from medical schools and later gone on to be the best and brightest medical students in their class. If medical school is your goal in life, you must persevere, but consider carefully all of your other options.

PUBLICATIONS

Allied Health Education Directory, 19th Edition. 1991. Order No. OP417591. American Medical Association, P.O. Box 2964, Milwaukee, Wisconsin 53201.

ECFMG Annual Report 1989. Free. Educational Commission for Foreign Medical Graduates, 3624 Market Street, Philadelphia, Pennsylvania 19104-2685.

Federal, State, and Private Activities Pertaining to U.S. Graduates of Foreign Medical Schools. September 27, 1985. Free. Document GAO/HRD-85-112. Government Accounting Office Documents, P.O. Box 6015, Gaithersburg, Maryland 20877.

Fenninger, L.D., "Foreign Medical Graduates in the United States: Policies and Attitudes." *Journal of Medical Practice Management,* 1 (No. 4): 275–281, April 1986.

Graettinger, J.S., "Datagram: Results of the NRMP for 1986." *Journal of Medical Education,* 61:617–619, July 1986.

Iglehart, J.K., "Reducing Residency Opportunities for Graduates of Foreign Medical Schools." *New England Journal of Medicine,* 313 (No. 13): 831–836, September 26, 1985.

"Quality of Preparation for the Practice of Medicine in Certain Foreign-Chartered Medical Schools." (Supplement) *Journal of Medical Education,* 56:963–979, November 1981.

Swanson, A.G., "How We Subsidize 'Offshore' Medical Schools." *New England Journal of Medicine,* 313 (No. 14): 886–888, October 3, 1985.

ORGANIZATIONS

American Association of Colleges of Pharmacy, 1426 Prince Street, Alexandria, Virginia 22314.

American Association of Colleges of Podiatric Medicine, 1350 Piccard Drive, Suite 322, Rockville, Maryland 20850.

American Society of Allied Health Professions, Suite 700, 1101 Connecticut Avenue, N.W., Washington, D.C. 20036.

Association of Physician Assistant Programs, Suite 300, 1117 North 19th Street, Arlington, Virginia 22209.

Association of Schools and Colleges of Optometry, Suite 690, 6110 Executive Boulevard, Rockville, Maryland 20852.

Association of Schools of Public Health, Suite 404, 1015 15th Street, N.W., Washington, D.C. 20005.

Association of University Programs in Health Administration, Suite 503, 1911 North Fort Myer Drive, Arlington, Virginia 22209.

Division of Baccalaureate and Higher Degree Programs, 10 Columbus Circle, New York, New York 10019.

MSKP. Section for Student Services. Association of American Medical Colleges, 2450 N Street N.W., Washington, D.C. 20037-1127

United Nations Bookshop, Room G.A. 32B, 405 East 42nd Street, New York, New York 10017.

POST-BACCALAUREATE PROGRAMS

For current list, write to: Health Pathways, 1600 Ninth Street, Room 441, Sacramento, California 95814–6422.

Current Programs

CALIFORNIA

Roberto Paez, Program Coordinator
Office of the Dean
UC Davis School of Medicine
Davis, CA 95616
916-734-7012

Eileen Munoz
Student Affairs Officer
UCI College of Medicine
E108 Medical Sciences I
Irvine, CA 92717

Karen A. Scheiber, Assistant Director
Special Admissions Support Program
CSD School of Medicine
Medical Training Facility, Rm. 162
La Jolla, CA 92093
619-534-4170

Dr. Edna Mitchell
Director, Graduate Studies
Post-Bacc Pre-Med Program
Mills College
Oakland, CA 94613
415-430-3309

FLORIDA

Suzette Rygiel, Co-chair
University of Miami, Coral Gables
College of Arts & Sciences
P.O. Box 248004
Coral Gables, FL 33124
305-284-5176

ILLINOIS

Vera Felts, Admissions Coordinator
MEDREP
Southern Illinois University, Carbondale
School of Medicine
Wheeler Hall
Carbondale, IL 62901
618-536-6671

MARYLAND

Dr. Carl E. Peterson
Department of Biological Sciences
Towson State University
Towson, MD 21204
301-830-3042

MASSACHUSETTS

Sylvia S. Field
Program Director
Health Careers Program
Harvard University Extension School
51 Brattle Street
Cambridge, MA 02138
617-495-2926

MICHIGAN

Dr. Wanda D. Lipscomb
Prematriculation Programs
College of Human Medicine
Michigan State University
A254 Life Sciences Bldg.
East Lansing, MI 44824-1317
517-353-5440

NEBRASKA

John T. Elder, Ph.D.
Department of Pharmacology
School of Medicine
Creighton University
Omaha, NE 68178-0225
402-280-3185

NEW YORK

Barbara L. Tischler
Director of Preprofessional Programs
405 Lewisohn Hall
Columbia University
New York, NY 10027
212-854-2881

Cathy Hadley-Samia
New York University
College of Arts and Sciences
Prehealth Advising Office
100 Washington Square East
Rm. 904, Main Bldg.
New York, NY 10003
212-998-8160

OHIO

Martha E. Sucheston, Ph.D.
Director, MEDPATH
MEDPATH-Medical Careers Pathway
The Ohio State University
College of Medicine
1072 Graves Hall
333 West 10th Ave.
Columbus, OH 43210
614-292-3161

PENNSYLVANIA

Gale Lang, Assistant Dean
Division of Special Studies
Bryn Mawr College
Bryn Mawr, PA 19010
215-526-7350

Katherine Pollack, Vice Dean
University of Pennsylvania
210 Logan Hall/CN
Philadelphia, PA 19104-6384
215-898-4847

CHAPTER 20

MEDICAL SCHOOL

"In the beginning . . . "

Genesis

Congratulations! If you are reading this chapter you have probably been accepted to medical school and are beginning to ask, "What have I gotten myself into?" Although the answer varies among schools, most institutions provide a similar four-year format of instruction.

During the first two years you will receive the basic science portion of your medical training. Most students find these years to be the most rigorous and demanding of their lives.

THE BASIC SCIENCES

Freshman Year

Freshman year of medical school typically involves courses in gross anatomy, histology, embryology, neuroanatomy, genetics, biochemistry, physiology, and behavioral science. Courses in medical ethics and legal medicine are often included in the first-year curriculum. As a rule, you will be in class from 8 A.M. to 5 P.M., Monday through Friday. The following gives a fairly accurate picture of what lies ahead.

Gross Anatomy. Gross anatomy is the study of the structures of the human body. Traditionally it is taught through lectures and dissection of a human cadaver. Every month you will study a new area of the body. The anatomy course is often divided into sections: head and neck, arms, legs, thorax, abdomen, back, perineum, and pelvis. Lectures usually last one or two hours, three to five times a week, for one or two semesters. Afternoons will be spent dissecting body parts covered in the lectures. Most students find gross anatomy their most interesting and most challenging course.

Histology.   Histology might better be called "microanatomy." It is the study of the cells that make up the human body. You will learn the location, type, and function of cells that are found throughout the body. Histology is usually taught three to five times per week in one-hour lectures and lasts one semester. At least one afternoon a week is spent in a histology lab looking at slides of body organs and tissue.

Embryology.   Embryology is the study of developmental anatomy. The course traces human cellular development from the sperm and ovum stage to the infant. Early in development, every structure of the human body comes from specialized cellular tissues, which develop into functional body parts. Often included in embryology are lectures on the drugs and diseases that can adversely affect embryo growth. You will learn what body part or organ system develops during each phase of the nine-month developmental process. Lectures will also cover attempts at preventing fertilization through the use of birth control devices. They are given three to five times per week, usually for one semester.

Neuroanatomy.   Neuroanatomy, the study of the central and peripheral nervous system, is the bane of many a medical student. Because of the many intricate nerve pathways that must be learned, most students find this one of their most challenging courses. It is usually a one-semester course that meets three to five times a week. A brain and spinal cord dissection lab also meets once a week.

Genetics.   Genetics is usually a one-semester course. Classes typically meet once or twice a week for an hour. Much of the course is spent learning to identify key features of children with genetic disorders. The class studies the many diseases caused by gene crosses and the consequences for the fetus.

Biochemistry.   Biochemistry is one of the "big three" courses taught to most freshman medical students, the other two being gross anatomy and physiology. Biochemistry is the study of chemical reactions that occur in the human body, examined on a cellular level. The ways in which these chemicals react to make organ systems function is also part of the course. The class often meets five times a week, one to two hours per day, for one or two semesters.

Physiology. Physiology is the study of the interaction of cellular systems and how they make the human body function. Topics covered include respiratory, kidney, cardiovascular (heart), and gastrointestinal function. The course meets one or two hours a day, five days per week, for one or two semesters.

Behavioral Science. Behavioral science is the study of how humans think and feel. Topics addressed might include how different races deal with pain, death, or birth. This class is usually limited, meeting one or two hours a week for one semester.

Ethics. Some schools require students to complete an ethics course and a legal medicine course. Ethics usually concentrates on such issues as euthanasia and abortion. Legal medicine covers the laws that affect the practice of medicine, such as malpractice laws. These courses usually meet one or two hours a week for one semester.

If the first-year curriculum seems as if it involves a lot of class time, it does. Medical school courses, in general, are not intellectually difficult, but the volume of material covered can be overwhelming. Most students consider themselves lucky to read textbooks once and notes twice before exams. Those students with the sharpest memorization and retention skills quickly rise to the top of any medical school class. Students with science backgrounds who have covered some or all of these courses also have an advantage. It is possible, however, to do well simply by studying a great deal, that is, 6 to 10 hours a day, seven days a week.

Sophomore Year

Most students find the second year of medical school more interesting, as schools concentrate on classes in understanding, diagnosis, evaluation, and treatment of disease. Courses typically include pathology, clinical pathology, microbiology, pharmacology, and diagnostic examination and evaluation. Many schools allow students to see patients and do practice histories and physicals.

Pathology. Pathology, by definition, is the study of suffering. It examines why diseases arise and how they affect tissue change or growth in the human body. Topics covered in pathology courses include immunology, infectious diseases, environmentally induced diseases, heart and blood vessel diseases, respiratory system diseases, and organ systems such as the liver, pancreas, kidney, urinary tract, gastrointestinal tract, spleen, genitals, skin, breasts, nervous system, and musculoskeletal system. Pathology is usually considered the most important class in the second year. It involves two hours of lecture time, five days a week, for the entire year. Additional time may be spent in the afternoons studying specimens of diseased tissue.

Clinical Pathology.   An extension of pathology is clinical pathology. The course covers clinical interpretation of laboratory tests. Some schools offer this as part of pathology; others separate the two.

Microbiology.   A close cousin of pathology, microbiology covers many of the same topics. A typical microbiology course studies bacterial, parasitic, and viral infectious diseases—some already well known to you, such as strep throat. You will learn about the many varieties of strep throat and the complications that can occur as a result of the disease. You will also study the bacteria that cause diseases such as meningitis (brain and spinal cord infection) and cellulitis (skin infection). In addition, you will discover that having a "worm" infection means you have one of hundreds of parasites that infect the human body. A final aspect of the course covers viruses, which cause illnesses ranging from the common cold to AIDS. This class will study how viruses reproduce, infect, and transmit the diseases they induce.

You will also study some of the basics of treatment of these diseases. Microbiology meets at least one hour a day, five days a week, for the entire year. Afternoon labs are spent studying these disease-causing agents under both light and electron microscopes.

Pharmacology.   Pharmacology is the study of how drugs function and interact, and how they are used in the treatment of disease. This is one of the most practical courses you will take during your second year. It meets one or two hours per day for the entire year; most schools do not offer labs.

Clinical Diagnosis.   Most schools offer this course in the second year. Typically it teaches students to do histories and physicals (H & P) and to recognize many of the physical findings of disease. Often students will work with a physician who has them practice physical exam techniques on his or her patients. The course usually meets one or two hours a day. Lab time is spent with the doctor, learning history and physical exam skills.

Boards Part I.   At the completion of the second year, most institutions require students to take National Boards Part I, a comprehensive exam covering the course work studied in the first two years of medical school.

In many schools you must pass this exam to continue into the third year. Many residency programs will also look at these scores in evaluating applicants. If you thought the MCAT was tough, wait till you see this one! You will be reviewing 10,000 pages of graduate-level texts in the two to three weeks you will be given to prepare for this exam.

THE CLINICAL SCIENCES

The final two years of medical school are spent on clinical rotations in several specialties. This is when you first begin to experience the "art and science" of medicine. Two to three months into your senior year you will have to choose one of these clinical specialties as part of your long-term career plans. Although many doctors eventually change specialties, the first years of internship and residency were often decided upon early in their senior year of medical school.

Junior Year

The light at the end of the tunnel grows bright as you start your third year of medical school. After this point, it would be unusual not to complete your medical degree. Third year generally consists of five two-month rotations in surgery, obstetrics and gynecology, pediatrics, internal medicine, and psychiatry. The other two months are often devoted to electives and vacation time.

Surgery.   Surgical rotation usually consists of two months of general surgery. A general surgeon does operations on the abdomen and may also operate on other areas of the body such as the arms, legs, chest, breasts, and neck. While on surgery you will be responsible for doing histories and physicals on patients admitted to the hospital, writing daily orders for maintaining the patient's diet, and, most important, assisting the surgeons in the operating room.

At the student level you will soon learn to think of yourself as a "human retractor." As a surgical assistant you will be asked to hold retractors and pull organs and body fat out of the way so the surgeon can dissect, remove, or revise whatever organ he or she is working on. Not a particularly glamorous job, and a privilege for which you will be paying!

While the operation is going on, you will be reviewing your anatomy. Most surgeons enjoy quizzing medical students on obscure body parts that have long since escaped your memory banks. Besides the daily quiz sessions, you will spend every third or fourth night "on call" in the hospital. This means you will be awakened by the nurse every hour or so, all night long, to check an oozing wound, prescribe a sleeping pill, or renew an IV order that happened to run out at 3 A.M. You will also admit new patients who arrive at the hospital for next-morning surgery.

Despite your lack of sleep, the next day you will be expected to stay awake in the operating room holding clamps and answering questions. And, despite chronic sleep deprivation, you will spend most of your "free" time reading surgical texts so you can pass the surgery exam at the end of the rotation. You will spend two to three afternoons a week in surgery clinic, seeing new patients or following up on those recovering from surgery.

Most students either love or hate surgery. The time demands are intense, but many students and doctors find the rewards of interesting and challenging surgery worth the mental and physical rigors.

Obstetrics and Gynecology.   Obstetrics and gynecology is often divided into two one-month rotations. You will spend one month doing gynecologic surgery, the other in obstetrics, delivering babies. The month in gynecology will be similar to your time in general surgery. You will be expected to assist in patient management, do admission histories and physicals, and help the surgeon in operations. Gynecologic operations include removal of the uterus and ovaries, operations on the vagina and bladder in elderly women who develop difficulty controlling urination, and the removal of tumors involving the reproductive organs. You will also assist in many dilatations and curettages (D and C's), a common operation to remove abnormal tissue lining the uterus.

Your month of obstetrics will involve assisting in the delivery of babies by either normal vaginal delivery or Caesarean section. In vaginal delivery your responsibility will be to check the mother for progression of labor, get the surgical tray ready in case special instruments such as forceps are needed, and awaken the obstetrician in time to deliver the baby. Just before the baby emerges, the surgeon will often make a small cut called an episiotomy to widen the cervix. After the baby is delivered, the mother will need the episiotomy sewn shut. As you get to know the surgeons you work with, they will let you do more and more of the delivery, including sewing the episiotomy closed. During C-section deliveries, you will again be the surgical assistant and hold clamps while the surgeon performs the operation to remove the infant. Near the end of your rotation in Ob/Gyn, you may be allowed to assist in closing the layers of fat, muscle, and skin of the C-section incision. During both of these months, in-hospital call will be every third to fourth night.

Pediatrics.   At most institutions, pediatrics is two months devoted to taking care of sick children in the hospital. Some schools allow time to see children in a clinic, perhaps one or two days per week. While on the pediatric service you will be on call every third to fourth night. Your responsibility will be to assist the intern or resident in admitting sick children to the hospital throughout the night. This often involves doing a history and physical and sometimes procedures such as a spinal tap to check for meningitis as a cause of the child's illness. While awake, you will spend your free time reading about your patients' problems and developing plans for helping them get over their illnesses. You will also help to care for patients who develop problems during the night.

In the morning you will make rounds on your patients with the intern, resident, and attending pediatrician. During rounds you will present your new patients to the attending doctor by giving him or her a brief summary of the key features of the H & P. You will be quizzed about your workup of each child's problem and your treatment plan. In your free time, you will prepare for your pediatric exam at the end of the rotation. If you like children, you will probably find this rotation interesting.

Internal Medicine.   For many students, the months of internal medicine will be some of the most intense of their medical training. This is the field of medicine that deals with medical problems in adults. Usually these problems occur in elderly patients with multiple medical conditions. Each day will begin early, usually around 6 A.M. You will start by making rounds on your patients, charting their progress, checking vital signs, ensuring their medicine orders are up-to-date, checking their IV fluids, and making sure, in general, that no complications occurred during the night.

Your rounds will be followed by rounds with the intern assigned to cover your patients, who will recheck them and make any adjustments he or she finds necessary. These rounds are followed by rounds with the senior medical resident. These are often quick rounds in which only the key features of each patient's problems are addressed. Finally, the patient's doctor appears and attending rounds begin.

The doctor will question you about your treatment of the patients and check their progress. He or she will also indicate physical exam findings you may have missed. Rounds usually last most of the morning. When they are complete, you will spend the afternoon looking up lab values, performing procedures on your patients, and making sure all diagnostic tests are complete. You may also have to attend a medicine clinic and see outpatients one or two afternoons per week. Assuming all is well, you can now go home for the day.

Every third or fourth night you will be on call. You will be responsible, along with the intern and the chief resident, for admitting patients to the hospital. As a new patient arrives, you will complete a history and physical and develop a treatment plan, which will be reviewed by the intern and resident. You rarely get to sleep, as new patients are always arriving and your patients already in the hospital will require supervision as new problems develop. In your few minutes of free time, you will be reading your medicine text in preparation for morning rounds.

The next day, your attending physician will have you present the histories and physicals of the patients you admitted the previous night. Internists are obsessive-compulsive people, and they will expect to have no facts missed. You will have to know the reason each patient is currently being hospitalized, the patient's medical history, all drugs the patient is now taking, and the patient's allergies, social history, family history, and surgical history, and to have made a detailed and complete physical exam. You will outline the possible causes of the patient's problems, how you plan to evaluate them, any test results available, and your treatment plan. As you make this presentation, you will frequently be interrupted with questions about the items you are outlining. Keep in mind that you have been up all night, admitted at least five patients, and probably will have a difficult time remembering these new patients, to say nothing of being able to answer questions about your management of their problems.

Psychiatry.   Psychiatry is usually a more laid-back rotation than most of the others in your third year of medical school. As with the others, you will take call every third or fourth night. Each day and call night you will be responsible for doing histories, physicals, and psych evaluations, specialized exams that assist in the diagnosis of psychiatric disease. Generally, the next day you will present your patients to your attending psychiatrist and resident. With them you will develop a treatment plan and monitor your patients' progress. You may also spend a few afternoons a week seeing outpatient clinic patients to monitor their home therapy and progress.

Senior Year

Electives. The fourth year of medical school is generally all electives. That is, you may do additional rotations in the specialties already covered or electives in many other specialty fields of medicine, including aerospace medicine, allergy and immunology, anesthesiology, pathology, cardiology, neurology, child psychiatry, critical care, preventive medicine, dermatology, radiology, emergency medicine, endocrinology, family practice, gastroenterology, geriatrics, hematology, infectious disease, oncology, neonatology, nephrology, neurosurgery, nuclear medicine, occupational medicine, ophthalmology, orthopedic surgery, otolaryngology, plastic surgery, pulmonology, radiation oncology, rheumatology, thoracic surgery, urology, and vascular surgery. Each of these specialties will be discussed in detail in the following chapter.

Matching. By September of your senior year, you will have determined the specialty you plan to pursue. You will begin to fill in applications for residency training programs. Starting in October and ending in February, you will take days off to travel across the United States interviewing for positions. In February you will send a list of the residency training programs that interest you, ranked in order of preference, to a national computer matching service. At the same time, the residency programs will turn in a list of the candidates they are interested in, also ranked in order of preference. In March or April, a computer will match you with the residency program that ranked you the highest and the one you ranked the highest. In other words, both you and the hospital training program will get your top mutual choice, your destiny being decided in a manner similar to a computer dating service.

Boards Part II. Near the end of your fourth year you will take Part II of the National Boards. This exam covers surgery, internal medicine, pediatrics, psychiatry, and obstetrics and gynecology. Some schools require passing this exam to graduate from medical school. Boards Part III is taken near the end of your internship. It covers clinical management of patients in the hospital.

Federal Licensing Exam (F.L.E.X.). Some schools will not require you to take boards. In these cases, you may elect to take the F.L.E.X. exam, a comprehensive board exam that covers all the material in Boards Parts I–III. This test is taken at the conclusion of medical school.

Virtually all states require you to pass either Boards Parts I-III or F.L.E.X. to obtain a medical license in the state. Residency programs also often use these tests to monitor your achievement.

Graduation

At the end of your senior year of medical school, you may be inclined to breathe a long sigh of relief. The medical degree you have received means little, however, until you have completed your internship, residency, and possibly a fellowship. Besides these, you will have to pass specialty board exams. Although you may now be called "Doctor," there is still a lot of time and effort you must devote to your education.

CHAPTER 21

RESIDENCY

**"To see patients without reading is like a ship
without a rudder; to read and not see patients is
like never having gone to sea."**

Sir William Osler, M.D.

Medical school provides the foundation of knowledge on which a physician builds his or her career, but it is in the subsequent years of internship and residency that the doctor learns the skills necessary to practice medicine. Residency training is spent at teaching hospitals throughout the United States and is comparable to an apprenticeship—although you may feel more like an indentured servant. You will be paid approximately $25,000 a year and will put in a 60- to 120-hour work week. Most interns and residents work seven days a week with rare weekends off.

You will also be on call every second, third, or fourth night, depending on your selected training program. For example, every third night on call means that you work from 6 A.M. Monday to about 6 P.M. Tuesday; Wednesday you work from 6 A.M. to 6 P.M.; Thursday from 6 A.M. to Friday 6 P.M.; Saturday 6 A.M. to 6 P.M.; and Sunday 6 A.M. to Monday 6 P.M. This cycle can continue for your entire three to seven years of training, depending on your specialty.

Every second night on call is a 126-hour work week; every third night on call is 114 hours; and every fourth night is 108 hours! Keep in mind that when another resident is sick or on vacation, you are often on call every second night.

INTERNSHIP

During your first year of training after medical school, you are called a "first-year resident" or "intern." Virtually all specialties require an internship. Some require a "rotating" internship or "transitional" year. This is similar to your third year of medical school; you will spend one to two months each doing surgery, internal medicine, pediatrics, obstetrics and gynecology, psychiatry, and one elective. You will also have three or four weeks of vacation time.

Other specialties will require your internship year to be more closely focused. For example, a first-year general surgery residency training program may require its first-year residents to spend six months doing general surgery and six months at assigned rotations in urologic surgery, thoracic surgery, plastic surgery, vascular surgery, and trauma surgery. An internal-medicine residency training program may require six months of general medicine caring for moderately sick patients in the medical intensive care unit, two months assigned to patients in the cardiac intensive care unit, and two months of electives such as neurology, hematology, cardiology, and oncology.

Generally, your first year of training demands the most time. Most residency training programs decrease the time commitment with each year of training; a few demand every third night on call for the entire training period. The average program requires interns to spend every third night in the hospital on call. This means being up all night admitting patients to the hospital, doing histories and physicals, writing admitting orders, teaching medical students, and taking care of patients' problems, which always seem to develop around 3 A.M. You will also be expected to work a full day after your on-call night.

After the internship year, you are a "resident" and no longer low man on the totem pole. In some programs you may continue every second, third, or fourth night on call; in others your call can decrease to a few nights a month. Some specialties require training in clinics or elective surgery during the day and do not involve treating patients who arrive during the night. Other residencies, such as radiology, have little or no direct patient care and will require only one resident in the hospital at night. Most radiologists' work is done during the day. Thus, if a hospital has 12 radiology residents, you may have to take call only every twelfth night, when your job may be to interpret the relatively few X-rays done at night.

Some residencies have home call. Dermatology emergencies are rare, so dermatology residents may take call from home or carry beepers and have to come in only a few times during their training. The majority of specialties, however, have patients in the hospital who develop complications at night or admit new patients during the night and require residents on the spot. A neurosurgery (brain surgery) resident's typical night may be spent attending several patients in a neuro intensive care unit, and when such a resident does get to bed at 2 A.M., he or she may be awakened by a call from the emergency-room physician. It seems another drunken motorcyclist has crashed and must be rushed to the operating room to have blood drained from his skull before the brain tissue is crushed and the patient dies.

As an intern or resident, you are never completely alone. Most hospitals have a hierarchy. For instance, every third night four pediatric interns may be on call. With them is one second- or third-year pediatric resident, who now takes call every fifth or sixth night. If a problem develops beyond the latter's capacities, the patient's attending (fully trained) pediatrician may be called at home to assist in solving the problem. Sometimes the attending pediatrician may come in from home to look at the patient and help decide on treatment. In more difficult cases, he or she may ask that a specialist be consulted to assist in diagnosis and treatment. For instance, if a child came in with a new heart murmur and the heart was no longer operating effectively, you might be asked to call in a pediatric cardiologist (heart specialist).

Medicine has many specialties. Some require several years of initial training in internal medicine, surgery, pediatrics, or psychiatry, followed by a fellowship in a more focused area. For instance, an oncologist is a doctor specializing in treating cancer. This specialist does a three-year residency in internal medicine or pediatrics followed by a three-year fellowship in oncology. Other specialties require an internship followed by two to three years of training. An emergency physician generally does a one-year rotating internship followed by three years of residency training in the emergency room. An anesthesiologist does an internship and three years of an anesthesiology residency.

The following details most of the residencies and fellowships available:

Anesthesiology

Internship plus three years of residency training. These doctors are responsible for putting patients to sleep during operations. Other than emergency surgery, they have no patient-care responsibilities at night. Call after the first year is infrequent, perhaps every fifth night. Fellowships are available in pediatric anesthesiology and critical care, each lasting one to three additional years.

Dermatology

Internship plus three years of residency training. These doctors diagnose and treat skin conditions. Their patient-care responsibilities at night are minimal and call is often taken from home. Fellowships are available in dermatopathology, which requires one or two more years.

Radiology

Internship plus three years of residency training. Radiologists interpret X-rays and perform specialized tests using radiographic equipment. They have little patient care at night. Call is usually in the hospital but as infrequently as three or four times a month. One- to two-year fellowships are available in ultrasound, CAT scan, MRI scan, nuclear medicine, and invasive radiology.

Emergency Medicine

Internship plus two to three years of residency training. These doctors specialize in treating emergencies in the emergency room. Rather than taking call, they work a set number of 8- to 12-hour shifts each month. One- to two-year fellowships are available in toxicology, pediatrics, emergency medical systems, and research.

Family Practice

Three years of residency training. Considered general practitioners, these doctors spend their years of training doing rotations in internal medicine, pediatrics, surgery, obstetrics and gynecology, psychiatry, radiology, orthopedics, critical care, and other electives. They learn to treat a wide spectrum of diseases and refer patients to specialists when their condition warrants. Call is usually every third to fourth night during internship and may decrease to every fifth or sixth night in the second and third years of training. One- to two-year fellowships are available in geriatric medicine (treating older patients), sports medicine, and obstetrics.

Internal Medicine

Three years of residency. These doctors specialize in the diagnosis and treatment of adult diseases. Because elderly adults tend to have more medical problems requiring hospitalization, many internists devote a significant part of their time to taking care of patients in the hospital in addition to busy office practices. Call is usually every third to fourth night for interns, decreasing to every fifth or sixth night in the final two years of training.

Many fellowships are available after three years of internal-medicine training. They generally last three to four years, with part of the time devoted to research. Cardiology fellows study patients with heart problems and do procedures such as echocardiograms and heart catheterizations. Critical-care fellows spend their training in medical intensive-care units. Endocrinology fellows learn specialized care of difficult-to-manage endocrine diseases such as diabetes. Gastroenterologists learn to treat diseases of the intestinal tract and learn specialized procedures, such as those in which fiber-optic scopes are used via mouth and rectum to examine the gastrointestinal tract. Fellows in geriatric medicine learn special skills needed to care for elderly patients. A hematology fellow studies the specialized care of patients with blood diseases such as hemophilia and cancers of the blood such as leukemia. Infectious disease fellows assist with the treatment of such complicated diseases as AIDS, tuberculosis, and meningitis. Nephrology fellows study patients with kidney problems and learn to manage patients undergoing dialysis. Oncologists take extra training in the treatment of cancers with chemotherapy. Fellows in pulmonary medicine specialize in diseases that infect the lungs, learning a special procedure in which a scope is put into the lungs through the mouth to take tissue specimens for diagnosis. Doctors learning to treat diseases that cause bone and joint breakdown do fellowships in rheumatology.

Thus, in addition to three years of demanding generalized internal medicine training, specialists devote additional years of training, taking call and working long days at relatively low pay, to develop the skills necessary to handle a narrow spectrum of patient problems.

Neurosurgery

Considered to be one of the most demanding surgical specialties, residency training in neurosurgery is typically six to seven years including internship. These doctors take call as often as every second to third night for seven years. Because of the delicacy of the operations performed, most being on the brain and spinal cord, the training is particularly rigorous. Residents attend neurosurgical emergencies, such as bleeding inside the skull from trauma, and remove tumors and aneurysms in brain tissue. There are no fellowships in neurosurgery.

Obstetrics and Gynecology

Ob/Gyn training begins with a one-year internship followed by a three-year residency. Call is every third to fourth night for most of the four years. These doctors learn to deliver babies, do Cesarean sections, and perform gynecologic surgery, such as removal of the uterus and ovaries, and tubal ligations. Fellowships are available in high-risk obstetrics, fertility, genetics, and oncology.

Ophthalmology

Ophthalmologists complete an internship followed by three years of surgical training. Eye emergencies are relatively few, so call is minimal after the internship and usually may be taken at home by carrying a beeper. These doctors do surgery on the eyes and prescribe eyeglasses. Fellowships are available in areas such as retinal repair and oncology.

Orthopedic Surgery

Orthopedic surgeons are "bone doctors" whose training consists of a general surgery internship followed by three to four years of orthopedic surgery. Orthopedists are frequently involved in the care of trauma victims and typically have a demanding call schedule of every third to fourth night for their four years of training. These specialists set bones, put on casts, and perform surgeries such as prosthetic hip replacements. Many also do an extra one or two years of fellowship training in specialties such as the hand, spine, oncology, sports medicine, and pediatrics.

Otolaryngology

Otolaryngologists are also known as ear, nose, and throat surgeons. Training consists of at least one year of general surgery followed by four years of ENT surgery. Call is generally every third to fourth night for five years. These doctors repair injuries to the ear, nose, and throat, as well as removing tumors, doing sinus draining procedures, and revising congenital abnormalities such as repairing a child's deformed lip or mouth. Fellowships are available in areas such as pediatrics and oncology.

Pathology

Pathologists study diseased tissue by viewing microscopic tissue specimens removed during surgery or autopsy. They are also responsible for all the laboratory tests hospital lab technicians perform. Pathologists usually follow a one-year internship with four years of pathology training. After the first year, few pathology programs require in-hospital call. Many pathologists do fellowships, and a number of one- to two-year fellowships are available.

Blood bank pathologists study blood used in transfusions. Chemical pathologists study tests evaluating chemical exposure to drugs and hazardous chemicals and become experts in laboratory tests. Dermatopathologists study diseases affecting the skin. Forensic pathologists do autopsies and assist police departments in looking for clues in the bodies of homicide victims. Hematologists study diseases affecting the blood, such as leukemia and sickle cell anemia. Immunopathologists study diseases of the immune system. Pathologists in microbiology learn about infectious diseases and their effect on human tissue. Radioisotopic pathologists study laboratory tests that use isotopes in diagnosing disease.

Pediatrics

Pediatricians treat children. Training involves a three-year residency and call is every third or fourth night. Pediatricians may do a number of two-year fellowships in areas such as cardiology, where they learn to treat children with heart problems. Pediatric endocrinologists treat children with diseases such as diabetes. Pediatric hematologists and oncologists treat children with blood diseases and cancer. Nephrologists treat children with diseases affecting the kidneys. Pediatric geneticists diagnose children with genetic diseases. Pediatricians in emergency medicine fellowships work in pediatric emergency rooms.

Physical Medicine and Rehabilitation

Training in physical medicine and rehabilitation usually lasts four years, one year of internship and three years of residency. Call may be every third to fourth night. These doctors care for patients recovering from accidents or debilitating diseases such as strokes. They also often assist in directing physical therapists in devising exercises for patients.

Plastic Surgery

Training in plastic surgery occurs in one of two ways. Most plastic surgeons complete a five- to six-year residency in general surgery, followed by a two-year residency in plastic surgery. A few programs allow residents to complete two years of general surgery followed by three years of plastic surgery. Plastic surgeons generally take call every third or fourth night for most of their training. These doctors perform many kinds of operations, including scar revision, breast enlargement and reduction, and face lifts. They may do fellowships in specialties such as hand surgery and microvascular surgery.

Preventive Medicine

Physicians in this field spend their careers in intervention in health and disease processes in communities and defined population groups. They work to increase behaviors that prevent disease and injury, and aim at early diagnosis and treatment. Training lasts two to three years including a one-year internship. Subspecialization is available within preventive medicine in fields such as aerospace medicine, occupational medicine, and public health.

Psychiatry

Psychiatrists care for the mentally ill and patients suffering from diseases such as depression, schizophrenia, and manic-depression. Training includes a one-year internship followed by a four-year residency. Call usually decreases to a few times a month as residents progress. A two- to three-year fellowship may be completed in child psychiatry. Also available is a fellowship in forensic psychiatry, which trains psychiatrists to care for patients deemed criminally insane.

Radiation Oncology

Radiation oncology requires a one-year internship followed by a four-year residency. Very few medical emergencies require the immediate attention of a radiation oncologist, and these doctors typically take call from home. They treat cancer patients with radiation, in some cases attempting to cure the patient, in others simply to slow down the disease's progression and decrease pain. Radiation oncology has few fellowships, and most involve extra training in research.

Surgery

Training in general surgery is demanding; residency usually requires five to seven years. Call may be every second to fifth night for all those years. These doctors do many surgical procedures on the abdomen, breasts, and extremities, and are trained to care for trauma victims. Many fellowships, usually lasting two to four years, are available after general surgery training. Colon and rectal surgery fellowships train doctors to do the more challenging operations on the lower bowel. Hand surgery fellowships develop skills in repairing hand injuries. Pediatric fellowships offer training in operating on small children. Plastic surgery fellowships supply training in specialized plastic surgery techniques. A thoracic surgeon may be trained to repair heart valves and do heart bypasses. Fellowships are also available in treating burn victims.

General surgeons may also do fellowships to become transplant surgeons of the pancreas, liver, and kidneys. Vascular surgeons receive training in operating on blood vessels and do procedures such as repairing abdominal aortic aneurysms. Surgeons may become critical care specialists who take care of very sick surgery patients in intensive care units. Many basic general surgery skills can be acquired in the first five or six years of residency, but the advanced skills, which allow doctors to do difficult, highly specialized operations, require additional training time.

Urology

Urologists operate on the urethra, penis, testicles, bladder, and kidneys. They perform operations to remove tumors and to repair traumatic injuries and dysfunctional organs. Training includes two years of general surgery followed by three years of urologic surgery. Fellowship training is available in pediatrics and oncology.

CONCLUSION

As you can see, the road to becoming a fully trained physician is long and arduous. Being on call several times a week is hard on you and your family. Spouses and children may find it difficult to accept the demands on your time from the hospital and your fatigue when you are at home. Additionally, most of your free time must be spent reading and studying textbooks and journal articles that help you learn the skills required of a specialist. Despite great sacrifices, in the end most doctors feel the reward of their work is the accomplishment of a lifelong dream.

CHAPTER 22

GOALS, PRIORITIES, AND CONCLUSIONS

"Press on: Nothing in the world can take
the place of persistence.
Talent will not; nothing is more common
than unsuccessful men with talent.
Genius will not; unrewarded genius
is almost a proverb.
Education alone will not; the world is
full of educated derelicts.
Persistence and determination alone
are omnipotent."

Calvin Coolidge

Getting into medical school is a difficult process. It involves much more than studying. You must be a good student, but you must also have qualities that allow you to negotiate a system designed to be selective. After reading this book, you should be aware that much of the selection process for medical school is arbitrary and capricious. Grades and MCAT scores are not the only selection criteria. Like it or not, the personality you display may make the difference between acceptance and rejection.

Having concluded that getting into medical school is as much an art as a science, you are ready to discover the true nature of the medical profession. Medicine demands that you be a student for the rest of your life. It is not without sacrifice. You must be willing to put your patients' interests before your own. You must be persistent. Many patients present a difficult diagnosis, and only through diligence will the etiology of the patient's illness be discovered. Hard work should not be something you fear, as the hours of a physician are long and arduous.

As you progress through your premedical training, do not be afraid of a difficult course if it will help you learn something that will make you a better physician. Delaying a difficult class may be appropriate in playing the "game" of getting into medical school, but never purposely select an easy instructor when a better instructor is available. Do not be afraid to face a challenge that, although difficult, provides you a superior learning opportunity. If you have the passion and energy to be a physician, no course should present a problem if you give it your best effort.

Keep your priorities straight. Premedical training is an opportunity to learn study skills that will help you become a good medical student and physician. Social activities are of equal importance, as the job of a physician demands that you understand and relate to people from all walks of life. Remember, the human qualities that make a good physician cannot be found in any textbook. You must get out and learn them!

THREE REQUIRED BOOKS

Carnegie, Dale. *How To Win Friends and Influence People.* Pocket Books, 1994 Reissue Edition.

Lazarus, Arnold, Ph.D., and Allen Fay, M.D. *I Can If I Want To.* Warner Books, 1977.

Ringer, Robert J. *Looking Out For Number One.* Fawcett Crest Books, 1977.

BEST OF LUCK IN YOUR MEDICAL CAREER!

If you have questions, comments, or suggestions, write:
Scott Plantz, M.D., Suite 103, 4450 Gulf Blvd., St. Pete Beach, FL 33706, or e-mail splantz@emedicine.com

For a response, please include a stamped self-addressed envelope.

ACCREDITED U.S. MEDICAL SCHOOLS

ALABAMA

University of Alabama
School of Medicine
Birmingham, AL 35294-0019
205-934-2330

University of South Alabama
College of Medicine
Mobile, AL 36688-0002
334-460-7176

ARIZONA

University of Arizona
College of Medicine
Tucson, AZ 85724
602-626-6214

ARKANSAS

University of Arkansas for
Medical Sciences
College of Medicine
4301 West Markham Street
Little Rock, AR 72205-7199
501-686-5354

CALIFORNIA

Loma Linda University
School of Medicine
Loma Linda, CA 92350
909-824-4467

Stanford University School of
Medicine
851 Welch Road, Room 154
Palo Alto, CA 94304-1677
415-723-6861

University of California, Davis
School of Medicine
Davis, CA 95616
916-752-2717

University of California, Irvine
College of Medicine
Irvine, CA 92717-3952
714-824-5388

University of California,
   Los Angeles
UCLA School of Medicine
Center for Health Sciences
Los Angeles, CA 90095-1720
310-825-6081

University of California,
   San Diego
School of Medicine
9500 Gilman Drive
La Jolla, CA 92093-0621
619-534-3880

University of California,
   San Francisco
School of Medicine
San Francisco, CA 94143
415-476-4044

University of Southern California
School of Medicine
1975 Zonal Avenue
Los Angeles, CA 90033
213-342-2552

COLORADO

University of Colorado
School of Medicine
4200 E. 9th Avenue, C-297
Denver, CO 80262
303-270-7361

CONNECTICUT

University of Connecticut
School of Medicine
263 Farmington Avenue,
   Rm. AG-062
Farmington, CT 06030-1905
203-679-2152

Yale University
School of Medicine
367 Cedar Street
New Haven, CT 06510
203-785-2696

DISTRICT OF COLUMBIA

George Washington University
2300 I Street, NW
Washington, D.C. 20037
202-994-3506

Georgetown University
School of Medicine
3900 Reservoir Road, NW
Washington, D.C. 20007
202-687-1154

Howard University College of
   Medicine
520 W Street, NW
Washington, D.C. 20059
202-806-6270

FLORIDA

University of Florida
College of Medicine
Box 100215
J. Hillis Miller Health Center
Gainesville, FL 32610
904-392-4569

University of Miami
School of Medicine
P.O. Box 016159
Miami, FL 33101
305-547-6791

University of South Florida
College of Medicine
12901 Bruce B. Downs
    Boulevard, Box 3
Tampa, FL 33612-4799
813-974-2229

GEORGIA

Emory University
School of Medicine
Administration Building
Atlanta, GA 30322-4510
404-727-5660

Medical College of Georgia
School of Medicine
Augusta, GA 30912-4760
706-721-3186

Mercer University
School of Medicine
Macon, GA 31207
912-752-2542

Morehouse School of Medicine
720 Westview Drive, SW
Atlanta, GA 30310-1495
404-752-1650

HAWAII

University of Hawaii
John A. Burns School of
    Medicine
1960 East-West Road
Honolulu, HI 96822
808-956-5446

ILLINOIS

Finch University of Health
    Sciences
Chicago Medical School
3333 Green Bay Road
Chicago, IL 60064
708-578-3206/3207

Loyola University Chicago
Stritch School of Medicine
2160 South First Avenue
Maywood, IL 60153
708-216-3229

Northwestern University
Medical School
303 East Chicago Avenue
Chicago, IL 60611
312-503-8206

Rush Medical College of Rush
    University
600 South Paulina Street
Chicago, IL 60612
312-942-6913

Southern Illinois University
School of Medicine
P.O. Box 19230
Springfield, IL 62794-9230
217-524-0326

University of Chicago
Pritzker School of Medicine
924 East 57th Street
Chicago, IL 60637
312-702-1939

University of Illinois
College of Medicine
808 South Wood Street
Chicago, IL 60612-7302
312-996-5635

INDIANA

Indiana University
School of Medicine
Fesler Hall 213
120 South Drive
Indianapolis, IN 46202-5113
317-274-3772

IOWA

University of Iowa
College of Medicine
100 Medicine Administration
   Building
Iowa City, IA 52242-1101
319-335-8052

KANSAS

University of Kansas School of
   Medicine
3901 Rainbow Boulevard
Kansas City, KS 66160-7301
913-588-5245

KENTUCKY

University of Kentucky
College of Medicine
Chandler Medical Center
800 Rose Street
Lexington, KY 40536-0084
606-323-6161

University of Louisville
School of Medicine
Health Sciences Center
Louisville, KY 40292
502-852-5193

LOUISIANA

Louisiana State University
School of Medicine in New
   Orleans
1901 Perdido Street
New Orleans, LA 70112-1393
504-568-6262

Louisiana State University
School of Medicine in Shreveport
P.O. Box 33932
Shreveport, LA 71130-3932
318-675-5190

Tulane University
School of Medicine
1430 Tulane Avenue, SL67
New Orleans, LA 70112-2699
504-588-5187

MARYLAND

Johns Hopkins University
School of Medicine
720 Rutland Avenue
Baltimore, MD 21205-2196
410-955-3182

Uniformed Services University of
the Health Sciences
F. Edward Hebert School of
Medicine
Admissions Office
Room A-1041
4301 Jones Bridge Road
Bethesda, MD 20814-4799
301-295-3101

University of Maryland
School of Medicine
655 West Baltimore Street
Baltimore, MD 21201
410-706-7478

MASSACHUSETTS

Boston University
School of Medicine
80 East Concord Street
Boston, MA 02118
617-638-4630

Harvard Medical School
25 Shattuck Street
Boston, MA 02115-6092
617-432-1550

Tufts University
School of Medicine
136 Harrison Avenue, Stearns I
Boston, MA 02111
617-636-6571

University of Massachusetts
Medical School
55 Lake Avenue, North
Worcester, MA 01655
508-856-2323

MICHIGAN

Michigan State University
College of Human Medicine
East Lansing, MI 48824-1317
517-353-9620

University of Michigan
Medical School
M4130 Medical Science I
Building
Ann Arbor, MI 48109-0611
313-764-6317

Wayne State University
School of Medicine
540 East Canfield
Detroit, MI 48201
313-577-1466

MINNESOTA

Mayo Medical School
200 First Street, SW
Rochester, MN 55905
507-284-3671

University of Minnesota—Duluth
School of Medicine
10 University Drive
Duluth, MN 55812
218-726-8511

University of Minnesota Medical
School—Minneapolis
Box 293-UMHC
420 Delaware Street, S.E.
Minneapolis, MN 55455-0310
612-624-1122

MISSISSIPPI

University of Mississippi
School of Medicine
2500 North State Street
Jackson, MS 39216-4505
601-984-5010

MISSOURI

Saint Louis University
School of Medicine
1402 South Grand Boulevard
St. Louis, MO 63104
314-577-8205

University of Missouri—
    Columbia
School of Medicine
One Hospital Drive
Columbia, MO 65212
314-882-2923

University of Missouri—
    Kansas City
School of Medicine
2411 Holmes
Kansas City, MO 64108
816-235-1870

Washington University
School of Medicine
660 South Euclid Avenue
    #8107
St. Louis, MO 63110
314-362-6857

NEBRASKA

Creighton University
School of Medicine
2500 California Plaza
Omaha, NE 68178
402-280-2798

University of Nebraska
College of Medicine
Room 4004, Conkling Hall
600 South 42nd Street
Omaha, NE 68198-4430
402-559-4205

NEVADA

University of Nevada
School of Medicine
Mail Stop 357
Reno, NV 89557
702-784-6063

NEW HAMPSHIRE

Dartmouth Medical School
    Admissions
7020 Remsen, Room 306
Hanover, NH 03755-3833
603-650-1505

NEW JERSEY

University of Medicine and
    Dentistry of New Jersey
New Jersey Medical School
185 South Orange Avenue
Newark, NJ 07103
201-982-4631

University of Medicine and
Dentistry of New Jersey
Robert Wood Johnson Medical
School
675 Hoes Lane
Piscataway, NJ 08854-5635
908-235-4576

NEW MEXICO

University of New Mexico
School of Medicine
Basic Medical Sciences Building,
Room 107
Albuquerque, NM 87131-5166
505-277-4766

NEW YORK

Albany Medical College
47 New Scotland Avenue
Albany, NY 12208
518-262-5521

Albert Einstein College of
Medicine of Yeshiva University
1300 Morris Park Avenue
Bronx, NY 10461
718-430-2106

Columbia University
College of Physicians and
Surgeons
630 West 168th Street
New York, NY 10032
212-305-3595

Cornell University
Medical College
445 East 69th Street
New York, NY 10021
212-746-1067

Mount Sinai School of Medicine
of the City University of
New York
Annenberg Building
Room 5-04
One Gustave L. Levy Place
Box 1002
New York, NY 10029-6574
212-241-6696

New York Medical College
Room 127
Sunshine Cottage
Valhalla, NY 10595
914-993-4507

New York University
School of Medicine
P.O. Box 1924
New York, NY 10016
212-263-5290

SUNY at Buffalo
School of Medicine and
Biomedical Sciences
CFS Building, Room 35
Buffalo, NY 14214-3013
716-829-3465

SUNY Stony Brook School
of Medicine
Health Sciences Center
Level 4, Room 147
Stony Brook, NY 11794-8434
516-444-2113

SUNY Health Science Center
at Brooklyn
College of Medicine
450 Clarkson Avenue
Box 60M
Brooklyn, NY 11203
718-270-2446

SUNY Health Science Center at
  Syracuse
College of Medicine
155 Elizabeth Blackwell Street
Syracuse, NY 13210
315-464-4570

University of Rochester
School of Medicine and Dentistry
Medical Center Box 601
Rochester, NY 14642
716-275-4539

NORTH CAROLINA

Bowman Gray School of
  Medicine of Wake Forest
  University
Medical Center Boulevard
Winston-Salem, NC 27157-1090
910-716-4264

Duke University School of
  Medicine
Duke University Medical Center
P.O. Box 3710
Durham, NC 27710
919-684-2985

East Carolina University
School of Medicine
Greenville, NC 27858-4354
919-816-2202

University of North Carolina at
Chapel Hill
School of Medicine
CB# 7000 MacNider Hall
Chapel Hill, NC 27599-7000
919-962-8331

NORTH DAKOTA

University of North Dakota
School of Medicine
501 North Columbia Road
Box 9037
Grand Forks, ND 58202-9037
701-777-4221

OHIO

Case Western Reserve University
School of Medicine
10900 Euclid Avenue
Cleveland, OH 44106-4920
216-368-3450

Medical College of Ohio
P.O. Box 10008
Toledo, OH 43699
419-381-4229

Northeastern Ohio Universities
College of Medicine
P.O. Box 95
Rootstown, OH 44272-0095
216-325-2511

Ohio State University
College of Medicine
270-A Meiling Hall
370 West Ninth Avenue
Columbus, OH 43210-1238
614-292-7137

University of Cincinnati
College of Medicine
P.O. Box 670552
Cincinnati, OH 45267-0552
513-558-7314

Wright State University
School of Medicine
P.O. Box 1751
Dayton, OH 45401
513-873-2934

OKLAHOMA

University of Oklahoma
College of Medicine
P.O. Box 26901
Oklahoma City, OK 73190
405-271-2331

OREGON

Oregon Health Sciences
University
School of Medicine
3181 S.W. Sam Jackson
Park Road
Portland, OR 97201
503-494-2998

PENNSYLVANIA

Jefferson Medical College of
Thomas Jefferson University
1025 Walnut Street
Philadelphia, PA 19107
215-955-6983

Medical College of Pennsylvania
and Hahnemann University
School of Medicine
2900 Queen Lane Avenue
Philadelphia, PA 19129
215-991-8202

Pennsylvania State University
College of Medicine
P.O. Box 850
Hershey, PA 17033
717-531-8755

Temple University School of
Medicine
Suite 305, Student Faculty Center
Broad and Ontario Streets
Philadelphia, PA 19140
215-707-3656

University of Pennsylvania
School of Medicine
Edward J. Stemmler Hall
Suite 100
Philadelphia, PA 19104-6056
215-898-8001

University of Pittsburgh
School of Medicine
518 Scaife Hall
Pittsburgh, PA 15261
412-648-9891

RHODE ISLAND

Brown University
School of Medicine.
97 Waterman Street
Box GA 212
Providence, RI 02912-9706
401-863-2149

SOUTH CAROLINA

Medical University of South
  Carolina
College of Medicine
171 Ashley Avenue
Charleston, SC 29425
803-792-3281

University of South Carolina
School of Medicine
Columbia, SC 29208
803-733-3325

SOUTH DAKOTA

University of South Dakota
School of Medicine
414 East Clark Street
Vermillion, SD 57069-2390
605-677-5233

TENNESSEE

East Tennessee State University
James H. Quillen College of
  Medicine
P.O. Box 70580
Johnson City, TN 37614-0580
615-929-6221

Meharry Medical College
School of Medicine
1005 D.B. Todd Boulevard
Nashville, TN 37208
615-327-6223

University of Tennessee,
  Memphis
College of Medicine
790 Madison Avenue
Memphis, TN 38163-2166
901-448-5559

Vanderbilt University
School of Medicine
209 Light Hall
Nashville, TN 37232-0685
615-322-2145

TEXAS

Baylor College of Medicine
One Baylor Plaza
Houston, TX 77030
713-798-4841

Texas A&M University Health
  Science Center
College of Medicine
College Station, TX 77843-1114
409-845-7744

Texas Tech University Health
  Sciences Center
School of Medicine
Lubbock, TX 79430
806-743-2297

University of Texas
Houston Medical School
P.O. Box 20708
Houston, TX 77225
713-792-4711

University of Texas
Medical School at San Antonio
7703 Floyd Curl Drive
San Antonio, TX 78284-7701
210-567-2665

University of Texas
Medical School at Galveston
G.210, Ashbel Smith Building
Galveston, TX 77555-1317
409-772-3517

University of Texas
Southwestern Medical Center
   at Dallas
Southwestern Medical School
5323 Harry Hines Boulevard
Dallas, TX 75235-9096
214-648-2670

UTAH

University of Utah
School of Medicine
50 North Medical Drive
Salt Lake City, UT 84132
801-581-7498

VERMONT

University of Vermont
College of Medicine
E-109 Given Building
Burlington, VT 05405
802-656-2154

VIRGINIA

Eastern Virginia Medical School
   of the Medical College of
   Hampton Roads
721 Fairfax Avenue
Norfolk, VA 23507-2000
804-446-5812

University of Virginia
School of Medicine
Box 235
Charlottesville, VA 22908
804-924-5571

Virginia Commonwealth
   University
Medical College of Virginia
School of Medicine
MCV Station, Box 980565
Richmond, VA 23298-0565
804-828-9629

WASHINGTON

University of Washington
School of Medicine
Health Sciences Center
A-300
Seattle, WA 98195
206-543-7212

WEST VIRGINIA

Marshall University
School of Medicine
1542 Spring Valley Drive
Huntington, WV 25704
304-696-7312

West Virginia University
School of Medicine
Health Sciences Center
P.O. Box 9815
Morgantown, WV 26506
304-293-3521

WISCONSIN

Medical College of Wisconsin
8701 Watertown Plank Road
Milwaukee, WI 53226
414-456-8246

University of Wisconsin Medical
School
Medical Sciences Center
Room 1250
1300 University Avenue
Madison, WI 53706
608-263-4925